GROW HEALTHY BABIES

GROW HEALTHY BABIES

The Evidence-Based Guide to a Healthy
Pregnancy and Reducing Your Child's
Risk of Asthma, Eczema, and Allergies

MICHELLE HENNING &
VICTOR HENNING, Ph.D.

RUBINEN

GROW HEALTHY BABIES

The Evidence-Based Guide to a Healthy Pregnancy and Reducing Your Child's Risk of Asthma, Eczema, and Allergies

ISBN   978-1-5445-0780-4   *Hardcover*
            978-1-5445-0779-8   *Paperback*
            978-1-5445-0781-1   *Ebook*

FOR C.S.

CONTENTS

INTRODUCTION

HOW TO GROW HEALTHY BABIES

My husband and I truly complement each other—with our allergies.

Together, we manage to be allergic to almost everything. We're the dinner guests everybody fears. I get stomach cramps from gluten, oats, and almonds. A recent allergy test revealed that I'm also slightly allergic to eggs and dairy. I guess I'm lucky—if Victor accidentally eats eggs, his throat, tongue, and face swell up. Dairy gives him a stuffy nose and inflamed skin. Give him too much sugar, or deprive him of sleep, and he'll scratch his arms, legs, and neck until they're bloody. He has had eczema from birth: when he was a baby, his parents sometimes had to restrain his hands at night because he was scratching so much, and once had to call an ambulance because of a bad asthma attack. To this day, he has asthma, hay fever, and a dust allergy, which means he is never far from an inhaler or a sneeze.

If you looked at both Victor's and my history of chronic disease, you'd conclude that we're not the most likely candidates for having a healthy child. And yet, our daughter is now five years old and doesn't show any signs of eczema, asthma, or allergies. As a baby, she never even suffered a single nappy rash, and she has been able to eat every food we've introduced without any problems. She has never needed or received antibiotics, and she's never had anything worse than a mild cold or vomiting bug (and thankfully, those never lasted longer than half a day and a dozen towels). She's as healthy a kid as we could wish for. With this book, we want to empower you to achieve the same for your child—by using simple, common-sense strategies that have been proven to work in thousands of scientific studies.

My own health troubles started early. I was born prematurely, contracted an infection at the hospital, and was pumped full of antibiotics. As a child, I was always sick. I had recurring ear infections and suffered from candida. My doctor kept feeding me antibiotics like it was candy. I was allergic to just about everything that touched me. Any sort of cream, spray, or cosmetics on my skin would make me explode with hives. As a teenager, I also developed hay fever and asthma, followed by a generous helping of severe acne. The acne spread all over my face, my chest, my back, and my arms. In strictly Catholic Ireland, where I grew up, you couldn't easily buy contraceptives, and I didn't need to: my acne did the trick. I wouldn't let boys get near me; I was too self-conscious and ashamed of my skin. I always covered up in the nightclub to hide any sign of spots. I struggled with my health, my skin, my schoolwork, and depression.

It didn't occur to me back then that my diet could have anything to do with my allergies and skin problems. I thought my diet was fine. After all, my dad is a chef—he used to let me sit in the kitchen of our seaside fish restaurant in rural Ireland and watch him cook. He taught me a love of good food. Even so, in retrospect, I didn't always eat a very healthy diet at home. Money was always tight, and when my parents were working, my brother and I often had tinned spaghetti hoops and Angel Delight, a powdered ready-to-mix pudding, for dinner. I had a sweet tooth as well—our cupboard was always stocked with mini chocolate bars and cookies.

Then, in high school, we had to take a class on food science. To me, it felt like a revelation. I remember thinking: "So that's it? All this junk food I'm eating is why I'm sick all the time." It seems laughably obvious now, but everything suddenly clicked into place for me. I went to a nutritionist for more advice, and she put me on a sugar-free diet. Not knowing any better, I switched to using artificial sweeteners, but I still noticed a big difference in my acne when I cut out the sugar. That got me interested enough to keep reading and digging into the research.

I became the go-to person for my friends about healthy eating. Looking back, I realise I didn't have a clue! Well—at least I didn't hurt anyone. When I was in my early twenties, I went to college to study nutritional therapy at the Irish Institute of Nutrition and Health. Based on what I learned, I gradually changed my whole diet. I stopped having sugar or artificial sweeteners. If I wanted something sweet, I ate fruit. I ditched processed foods and switched to whole foods. I cut out gluten after finding out that it was linked to anxiety and mood swings in gluten-intolerant people. My acne cleared completely. My moods improved dramatically, and I went from being a volatile person, prone to anxiety and bursts of anger, to being more even-keeled.

I had additional good reasons to be thinking about diet and health. My mother was diagnosed with multiple sclerosis when

I was eleven. One of her brothers later died of the disease, and another developed Parkinson's disease. So did their mum—my grandmother. They all had grown up and lived on an idyllic farm in rural Ireland, playing outside while their father—unaware of the dangers—doused the field right next to them in pesticides. It was the 1950s, and pesticides were new; people had no idea about their long-term health risks. On my mother's side of the family, several of my cousins went on to suffer from ulcerative colitis and other health issues. Could it really just be genetics for this many members of the same family to develop autoimmune conditions? I doubted it.

After college, I went to live in Paris to pursue my dream of working as a singer-songwriter, but I also wrote a food blog and never lost my interest in nutrition. In October 2011, I was in Dublin to record a new album with my band. At the same time, my future husband, Victor, was there to attend a technology conference, and a mutual friend of ours invited me over to the nightclub where the conference afterparty was happening. That's where Victor and I met. We started talking, and I told him that I was working as a singer-songwriter but that I was a nutritionist by training. He quipped, "Oh, so what do you do—prescribe carrots?" I gave him a death stare. It dawned on him that we weren't off to a good start. The look of regret on his face was quite endearing, and we kept talking. Later, we left the nightclub and walked along St. Stephen's Green to meet a friend of mine. My skinny leather jacket was completely unsuitable for a cold November night, and I was freezing and rubbing my hands to warm them up. Victor noticed and, despite shivering himself, took off his gloves and offered them to me. I thought, *"Maybe this guy isn't so bad after all…"*

At the time, the stress of running his own company had made

his childhood eczema flare up badly. He had patches of raw, scaly skin on his arms and the backs of his knees, and his hands and neck would sometimes break out in blisters. While his stress and lack of sleep were bad, his diet was even worse. He lived on about fourteen microwave meals a week. He didn't have the faintest idea about how to cook anything and was completely ignorant of the link between diet and health. As we got to know each other, I told him he couldn't keep living like that—it was making his eczema worse, and it wasn't good for the rest of his health either. Because I still lived in Paris and he lived in London, I taught him how to cook over Skype. We started with really simple meals, like roasted chicken and sweet potatoes. He would text me pictures while cooking. Sometimes he was proudly showing off a green smoothie or a successfully cooked vegetable, but mostly it was "Is this what it's *supposed* to look like?"

Besides using inhalers for his asthma and hay fever, he had also been slathering himself in corticosteroid cream to manage his eczema. Changing his diet has made a huge difference—he has mostly stopped using the corticosteroid cream, his skin has cleared up, and his other allergies have also improved significantly. As a bonus, after eight years of practice, he has now become a really good chef, particularly cooking yummy Korean food.

Of course, food isn't the answer to everything. I suspected that his and my health problems were at least partly genetic. After we were married and thinking about starting a family, my doctor told me that—since we both had chronic health issues—our baby also had a 75 percent chance of developing eczema or allergies.[1] I thought, "There's no way I'm accepting this. There *has to be* a way to prevent our baby from inheriting our health problems."

Again, Victor and I truly complemented each other, but this time more productively than by making life difficult for dinner hosts. I had studied nutritional therapy but had spent the past five years working in music—so my scientific training and understanding of statistics had become a bit rusty. Victor knew nothing about nutrition and health, but he had just completed his PhD on the role of emotions in decision-making, had co-authored chapters in statistics textbooks, and published in leading academic journals. During his PhD studies, he had also founded a company called Mendeley. By the time we met, Mendeley had become the world's largest scientific collaboration platform, connecting millions of researchers around the globe.

Together, we started researching the link between diet, lifestyle, and chronic illness. We systematically combed the medical literature, determined to find out what we could do to *really* make a difference in our future child's health. In this book, I'll share with you what we found.

HOW THIS BOOK IS ORGANISED

In the remainder of this introduction, I want to briefly explain how the science of medicine generates the knowledge this book is based on. How do medical studies determine what "works" and really makes a difference to patients' health? If we talk about "reducing the risk" of a chronic disease, what do we mean?

In chapter 1, we'll begin by reviewing the chronic conditions this book aims to prevent: asthma, eczema, and allergies. What are they, what causes them, and how are they linked? Why are they on such an alarming rise all over the world?

Next, in chapter 2, we'll learn about the microbiome—the

friendly bacteria living in and on our bodies. We'll see how, beginning from birth, they shape your child's developing immune system and play a central role in the prevention of inflammation and chronic diseases. Understanding this is the key to unlocking the full potential of this book, because it underpins much of the science described in the subsequent chapters.

In chapter 3, we'll tackle the biggest threat to a healthy microbiome: antibiotics. As lifesaving as they can be, they are generally overprescribed and often unnecessary. We'll discuss why, when, and how to avoid them and possible alternatives before you resort to antibiotic treatment.

In chapter 4, we'll see how your diet is the steering wheel for your microbiome. What you eat influences the composition of bacteria in your gut—directly and immediately. We'll answer the question: which foods lead to a healthy microbiome? Chapters 5 and 6 zoom in on the subject of dietary fats and sugars—these dramatically impact the level of inflammation in your body, your overall health, and your child's development. Chapter 7 will show you the key nutrients for a healthy pregnancy and healthy baby. Many women are deficient in these nutrients, and we'll discuss the foods or supplements from which you can get them.

In the two chapters thereafter, you will see how certain purchasing and lifestyle choices affect your health and that of your child. Chapter 8 lays out the health benefits of choosing organic foods, and chapter 9 reveals the health risks associated with many cleaning products, cosmetics, and baby-care items. All too often, these are laden with chemicals linked to the development of chronic diseases, but you will see how to find healthier alternatives.

The last two chapters focus on birth and post-pregnancy choices.

Chapter 10 shows you the surprising ways in which the way your baby is born impacts its health—via birth hormones and the microbiome. In chapter 11, you will learn how breastfeeding shapes your child's health and cognitive development, and how it helps to prevent not just allergies but many other serious childhood diseases. We will also review how to get help if you are struggling with breastfeeding—like I did—or what formulas to choose if you are unable to breastfeed.

Finally, the summary chapter will pull it all together. Perhaps you are eager to know what you can do right away and what to prioritise. In that case, feel free to skip right to the end and read the summary—you can always go back and dive deeper into the previous chapters to learn more.

GAINING MEDICAL KNOWLEDGE

There are few things that are more confusing and frustrating than googling for health advice. The internet is full of contradictory anecdotes, conflicting advice, and weird wonder cures. If you want to find out how to prevent your baby from having chronic diseases, what can you do to cut through all of this noise?

Asking your family doctor or general practitioner (GP) for advice is certainly a good first step. Even better, there is a growing number of doctors who specialise in "integrative medicine"—that's the approach to medicine which takes into account a patient's lifestyle factors like nutrition, wellness, exercise, sleep, relationships, and mental health. You could also seek out a doctor who specialises in allergies (called an allergist).

Your next option is to go straight to the source of medical knowledge. New research is constantly advancing our understanding of how our child's immune system develops, how it interacts with the world around us, and what we can do to influence it in the right direction. You might be surprised to learn that much of this knowledge is freely available to the public in medical research databases. However, deciphering it requires traversing a maze of hard-to-understand "medicalese," surrounded by a thorny shrubbery of statistics. That's what Victor and I did, with the scrapes on our faces to prove it—you'll find more than 700 references to research papers in the appendix. The goal of this book is to take the latest medical evidence on how to prevent chronic diseases in children and summarise it in a way that's accessible and easy to understand, even if you have no medical or scientific training whatsoever.

Not all medical evidence is created equal, however. Some research papers are merely a collection of hypotheses that haven't yet been tested, others are anecdotal case studies based on a single patient, and yet others are rigorous experiments involving hundreds of patients. So let's take a moment to understand the three kinds of medical studies on which the information in this book is based: *observational studies, randomised controlled trials,* and *meta-analyses.*

What these three kinds of studies have in common is that the researchers compare *groups* of people, not just individual patients. Usually, the larger the number of people involved in the study (also called the "sample size"), and the larger the groups of people being compared, the better. What researchers are interested in when studying these groups are differences in health *outcomes*: whether the people in one group stayed healthy while the people in the other group got sick. More importantly, if there are differences in health outcomes, the researchers want to identify the underlying causes. These could be just about anything: something that one group does that the other group doesn't do (e.g., take a certain vitamin, breastfeed, smoke), or something that one group is exposed to that the other group isn't exposed to (e.g., a medical treatment, pesticides, environmental chemicals). These are the so-called risk factors (if they increase the risk of illness) or protective factors (if they lower the risk of illness).

If researchers design a study where they can control and manipulate these risk factors or protective factors, it's called a *randomised controlled trial* or *RCT*. The participants in the study are split into two groups. One group gets a treatment (or "intervention"), the other one doesn't. At the end of the study, the researchers compare the health outcomes between the two groups to see whether the treatment had an effect.

However, sometimes researchers aren't able to design such RCTs because it would be unethical, impractical (e.g., too expensive, too time-consuming), or impossible (e.g., due to limitations in medical technology). For example, it would clearly be very unethical—if not to say evil—to intentionally expose pregnant women to pesticides to see whether it harms their babies' health. In such a case, researchers instead identify pregnant women who were *coincidentally* exposed to pesticides by living near pesticide-sprayed fields, versus women who weren't. The women who were exposed to pesticides are called the "case group," and the women who weren't exposed are called the "control group." At the end of the study, the researchers compare the two groups to see whether the pesticide exposure made a difference to the babies' health. Studies like these are called *observational studies* and come in different flavours, like "cohort studies" or "case-control studies." The example above is a cohort study, which looks forward in time: the researchers start with a risk factor (e.g., exposure to pesticides), then compare the different health outcomes in the future. Case-control studies, on the other hand, look backwards in time: researchers start with a health outcome we see today (e.g., babies that developed asthma vs babies that didn't), then comb through the risk factors or protective factors in the past which could have caused this difference in health.

Both RCTs and observational studies have their respective strengths. RCTs are considered to produce stronger evidence than observational studies because researchers have greater control over the risk factors and protective factors. This makes it easier to demonstrate "causality," meaning whether a treatment or exposure actually causes a health outcome. Let's say you randomly assign people into two groups, A and B. If you then give a treatment to group A but only a placebo to group B, and group A is healthier than group B at the end of the study, you can be reasonably confident that it was your treatment that caused the difference. It's not that simple with observational studies: maybe any difference that you observed between groups was caused by a hidden risk or protective factor that you weren't aware of. But observational studies have a key advantage: they can involve a much larger number of people, over a much longer period of time—e.g., you could compare the medical records of everyone born in a country over the last century. Generally, the more people you can observe, the stronger your evidence.

There's yet another type of study that's interesting for us. What if you could combine the data from dozens, maybe even hundreds, of RCTs and observational studies into a single result? That's what a *meta-analysis* does. Researchers trawl through medical databases to find all previous studies on a given subject, identify the ones that are suitable for inclusion in the meta-analysis, then combine them into a single result using clever statistical methods. Many researchers consider meta-analyses to be the gold standard of medical evidence.

Yet, beyond the strength of the evidence, there is one more thing we need to consider: what the evidence actually tells us. Knowing that something is a risk factor, or a protective factor, is interesting. But what we really want to know is, *how big of a difference does it actually make*? In other words, *do I really need to care*? In medical research papers, this question is answered using the concept of "relative risk," and it's central to understanding the recommendations in this book. Let's look at a simple example.

Say we are interested in finding out whether taking antibiotics during pregnancy raises a child's risk of developing asthma later in life. Imagine a study finds that 25 percent of children exposed to antibiotics in the womb go on to develop asthma. The study also finds that when children are *not exposed* to antibiotics in the womb, the rate of asthma is only 12.5 percent. In other words, exposure to antibiotics in the womb *doubles* a child's risk of developing asthma. This ratio, which compares the risk between two groups, is what researchers call relative risk.[a]

Throughout this book, when we say "X increases the risk of asthma by 200 percent" or "Y decreases the risk of allergies by 50 percent," we are always referring to relative risk. If you

---

a   Depending on the type of study, the difference in risk can also be reported as an "odds ratio" or "hazard ratio." Those are technical details which we'll ignore in this book. For our purposes, it's enough to understand that hazard ratios are reasonably similar to relative risk, and that we can estimate relative risk from odds ratios using a bit of maths.[2] Whenever a study reported odds ratios, we converted it to relative risk using the ClinCalc. com converter tool.[3]

are interested in diving deeper into the concept of relative risk, there is a detailed example calculation in "Appendix 1: Understanding the Concept of Relative Risk and Absolute Risk."

A final note on wording before we move on. In everyday language, "risk," "probability," "chance," "odds," and "likelihood" are often used interchangeably. We'll do the same in this book. They don't mean the same thing in statistics, but—with due apologies to the statisticians among our readers—we'll go with the colloquial use and treat them as synonyms to make for less repetitive reading.

TAKING IT STEP BY STEP

Health is rarely all or nothing—it's a spectrum. Children aren't either just healthy or chronically ill. Even within chronic illness, there is a wide range of health outcomes. It makes a big difference whether your child suffers from occasional wheezing versus severe, life-threatening asthma; a mild food intolerance versus a severe allergy which will trigger anaphylactic shocks; being allergic to only one food versus a dozen different ones; and occasional dry, itchy skin patches versus constantly red-raw, inflamed skin all over your face and body.

As you will see in this book, you can influence where your child lands within this spectrum of health—and to a surprisingly large degree. However, some factors will remain outside of your control: genetics, economic and environmental circumstances, and pure luck. This small element of randomness means that your chain-smoking, fast-food eating friend could do everything "wrong" and still end up having a healthy baby. It's possible, but it's not very likely! It also means that you could be doing everything "right," and your child could still end up with an allergy. That's *also* possible, but fortunately it's *also* not very likely.

If you make healthy choices, your baby has a very good chance of being healthy. The medical evidence presented in this book suggests that you can reduce your child's risk of asthma, eczema, and allergies by as much as 90 percent, and those are pretty good odds.

What I hope you take away from this book is that every little bit helps. Whatever you can do for your child's health, given your circumstances, is worth doing. It doesn't matter when you start—before, early, or late in the pregnancy, even thereafter. It's never too late to make healthier choices. They will always be beneficial. If you think of health as a spectrum, each positive step you take will nudge your child's chances just a little bit further towards good health.

This also means that *if* you do make a few less-than-optimal choices, they are at worst a few steps backwards, not a catastrophe. Whether it's circumstances, a temporary lapse of willpower, or things in your past which you didn't know were harmful to your health—don't be too hard on yourself. It's not helpful to spiral into doomsday scenarios, as I'm sometimes guilty of doing, and worry that you might have blown your child's chances for good health. Dust yourself off and make healthier choices again the next day. It's a journey and a lifestyle, not something you do for a while until you're "done." I've studied nutrition and health since college, yet I'm still learning about and discovering things that could improve my health all the time.

Equally important, don't get overwhelmed by trying to do

everything at once. Just focus on an area where you feel you can make the biggest difference to your health and start there. It's not about perfection but making progress towards a healthier lifestyle for yourself and your children. Don't let the perfect be the enemy of the good. Every little bit helps.

Now, let's get started!

PART I

YOUR BABY'S DEVELOPING IMMUNE SYSTEM AND THE MICROBIOME

CHAPTER 1

THE RISE OF ATOPIC DISEASES AND ALLERGIES

Today, in many countries, your child is more likely to develop a chronic disease than to stay healthy. Conditions like asthma, eczema, allergic rhinitis, and food allergies (sometimes jointly called atopic diseases, though there are also non-atopic allergies) are on the rise everywhere you look. If you had walked into a random kindergarten or classroom anywhere in the world just forty years ago, you would be hard-pressed to find a single child with any of these health issues. Walk into that same kindergarten or classroom today, and up to half of the children in it will be affected by some form of atopic disease or allergy.

What's causing this seemingly unstoppable increase in chronic health problems starting from early childhood? That's the question we'll tackle in this chapter. Let's begin by briefly reviewing the chronic health issues we are aiming to prevent.

ASTHMA

An asthma attack can feel frightening. You strain and struggle to breathe, while an invisible band seems to tighten around your chest and in your throat. Asthma attacks can be triggered by exercise or stress, or by things in the environment: cigarette smoke, pollen, animal dander, mould, or dust mites. The underlying cause, however, is a chronic inflammation of the airways, or bronchi, in your lungs. The bronchi—a network of ever-smaller branching tubes which transport the air deep into your lungs—swell in response to irritants that your body believes to be a threat. The muscles around the bronchi tighten and your airways produce extra mucus. That is what causes breathing difficulties and wheezing.

Asthma is serious: every year, it kills 180,000 people. According to the World Health Organization, it is now the most common chronic disease in children worldwide.[4] It's also one of the leading reasons for children missing school days or being hospitalised.[5-7]

Globally, the number of people diagnosed with asthma has increased by 50 percent every decade. In Western Europe, twice as many people now suffer from asthma than just ten years ago.[8] Of course, this upwards trajectory in asthma also includes children. In the United States and across many European countries, about one in ten children will develop asthma.[9,10] In the United Kingdom, where Victor and I lived when we began trying for a baby, a child's risk is about one in four; in Australia, it is nearly one in three.[10,11]

Managing asthma symptoms usually combines long-term use of corticosteroid inhalers, which tone down the inflammation in the airways, with quick-relief medication in case of asthma attacks. The good news: the medical evidence in this book will show you how up to *nine out of ten* cases of asthma can be prevented by making certain diet and lifestyle choices.

ECZEMA

While asthma is potentially more serious—in that it could lead to hospitalisations or even death—eczema often has a bigger negative impact on your quality of life, as we can testify from our own experience. Having a bad eczema flare-up makes you want to crawl out of your skin, literally. It begins with an itch that gets worse the more you scratch it, to the point where you cannot stop yourself from clawing at your skin until it bleeds. The urge to scratch is overpowering, and no amount of willpower will stop you from scratching. When the damage is done, your skin feels raw and painful. It stings and burns. At worst, you can feel it oozing and sticking to your clothes. If the eczema flare-up is on your neck or in the crook of your arms and legs—these are the most common areas—it can hurt to turn your head or bend your limbs. It robs you of your sleep, and not necessarily just you but also those around you. As I type this, I'm bleary-eyed because Victor woke both me and our daughter at five o'clock this morning by scratching and tossing around in bed. Eating sugar late in the evening always does this to him, and yesterday at 10:00 p.m. he had some of his leftover chocolate birthday cake.

In addition to the physical burden, many kids feel ashamed of showing their patchy, scaly, blistered skin in public. I certainly felt that way, as did Victor and our friends who grew up suffering from eczema. It's particularly tough when you have an eczema flare-up on your face, or when other kids make cruel comments on how awful your skin looks. Studies show that if you have eczema, you are at a higher risk of developing anxiety and depression—and the more severe the eczema, the higher the risk.[12]

So what is eczema? Again, it's chronic inflammation—in this case, of the skin. The skin becomes dry, rough, reddened, and itchy. Like asthma, it is the result of an immune system gone haywire. Often, the underlying problem is an allergy, and avoiding the allergen can turn down the symptoms or even make them go away completely. An interesting recent discovery is that children with eczema have a different set of bacteria on their skin than healthy children, and this could open the door to exciting new treatment options. The standard treatments, however, are moisturizing lotions and corticosteroid creams. These can somewhat relieve the symptoms, but the corticosteroids come with nasty side effects if used long term.

Like asthma, eczema is on a rapid rise. In the United States, eczema rates have doubled since 2000,[13] now affecting about 10 percent of children. Across industrialised countries, the rate is between 10–20 percent[14]—and in some countries, like France, about 30 percent of children are affected.[15] The common wisdom is that most children with eczema eventually "outgrow" it. However, a study conducted by researchers at the University of Pennsylvania examined the health records of 7,157 children with eczema over a period of twenty-four years, starting at age two.[16] Even at age twenty-six, more than 80 percent of children still suffered from occasional eczema symptoms. The researchers concluded that eczema is probably a lifelong condition.

Moreover, eczema is frequently the beginning of the so-called atopic march: of the children with eczema, a majority go on to develop allergic rhinitis (the combined name for hay fever and dust allergy) or asthma, or both.[17,18] Yet, again I'm happy to say that the science in this book shows how certain diet and lifestyle choices could *prevent up to nine out of ten* cases of eczema.

ALLERGIC RHINITIS AND FOOD ALLERGIES

Allergy symptoms range from mildly annoying to life-threatening. They are a reaction of the immune system to a foreign substance called an allergen. These allergens—whether eaten, inhaled, or touched—are usually harmless, but the immune system perceives them to be a threat and launches an attack on the "invader." When it does, you might experience a wide range of symptoms:

- Itchy skin and eyes
- A runny nose and sneezing
- Skin rashes and hives
- Nausea, diarrhoea, and vomiting
- Wheezing, coughing, and asthma attacks
- Dizziness and low blood pressure

The most serious allergic reaction is called anaphylactic shock (or anaphylaxis) in which the immune system runs amok, triggering a rapid swelling of the throat and tongue, breathing difficulty, vomiting, and low blood pressure. Without emergency measures like epinephrine injections, anaphylaxis can be deadly.

Allergies have become so common that I couldn't believe the numbers when I first heard them. Across the United States and European Union (EU), 40–50 percent of *all children* are being diagnosed with an allergy, and by 2025, more than half the EU population is projected to be allergic.[19,20] Just take a moment to ponder this: half of all children born in these countries will grow up suffering from allergies, having to avoid harmless pollen or pets, or living in fear from life-threatening anaphylactic shocks. Hospital admissions from anaphylactic shocks have increased sixfold in the last twenty years.[21]

Hay fever and dust allergy (allergic rhinitis) are still the most common allergies, but food allergies have been catching up fast over the last twenty years as well. Previously rare, they are now called the second wave of the allergy epidemic, with the potential to develop into a "tsunami of allergic disease." Since the late 1990s, industrialised countries like the United States and UK have seen a threefold rise in food allergies—about 12 percent of kids are now expected to develop them.[22] In many countries, like Australia, hospitalisations due to food allergies have increased fivefold and referrals to food allergy doctors have increased tenfold.[23] Dairy and eggs are the most common food allergies in kids, followed by peanuts, soy, wheat, tree nuts (like walnuts and cashew), sesame, fish, and shellfish. Some kids will outgrow their allergies, but unfortunately peanut, tree nut, seed, and seafood allergies tend to be lifelong.[24]

As with asthma and eczema, the medical studies in this book describe ways to *prevent up to nine out of ten* cases of rhinitis and food allergies.

WHAT ARE THE CAUSES OF ATOPIC DISEASE?

What causes atopic diseases like asthma, eczema, and allergies, and how do we explain their rapid rise? For one, allergies run in families. If neither parent has an allergy, the child's risk of developing an allergy is around 10–20 percent. If one parent has an allergy, the risk rises to 50 percent; if both parents have allergies, the child has a 75 percent chance of becoming allergic.[1] However, genetics alone can't explain why atopic diseases are rising at such a rapid rate. Something else must be going on.

Atopic diseases have one thing in common: a hypersensitive immune system that is constantly on high alert, fighting supposed threats by triggering inflammation. But what makes the immune system become hypersensitive?

To understand, let's take a closer look at how the immune system identifies threats. This task falls to a group of immune cells known as T helper cells, or Th cells for short—think of them as police officers that patrol the body and keep on the lookout for intruders.

Th cells originate in the bone marrow and then undergo "police training" in the thymus, a small gland located in the chest. There, they are assigned to different "police units"—two of the most important ones are called Th1 and Th2. Each police unit has a specific task. Th1 cells patrol for bacteria and viruses that try to enter the body's cells. Th2 cells, on the other hand, hunt down parasitic worms and other parasites attempting to enter the bloodstream and bodily fluids.[25]

When one of these two police units becomes active and mounts an immune response against a threat, it "radios" the other unit to stand down and get out of its way. In medical language, Th1 and Th2 downregulate each other. It's like a seesaw—when Th1 activity goes up, Th2 activity goes down, and vice versa. After the threat has been neutralised, the seesaw returns to a balanced state. The cops can relax a little, so to speak. In healthy people, this is the normal state: Th1 and Th2 immune activity stay in balance, and neither is permanently active.

In people with chronic conditions, this isn't the case. The seesaw is out of balance because one of the two police units is always on high alert. When Th1 is permanently active, the immune system mistakes the body's own cells for bacterial invaders and attacks them. The results are autoimmune diseases like rheumatoid arthritis, inflammatory bowel disease, multiple sclerosis, type 1 diabetes, or lupus. Conversely, when Th2 is permanently active, the immune system mistakes food particles, pollen, dander, or other harmless objects for parasitic invaders and mounts an immune response. The results are atopic diseases like asthma, eczema, and allergies.[26,27]

Here's a little drawing to illustrate the principle:

Th1 vs Th2 immune activity

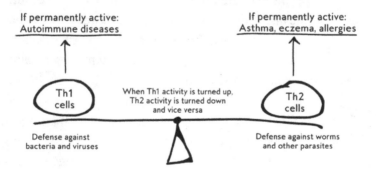

If permanently active:
Autoimmune diseases

If permanently active:
Asthma, eczema, allergies

Th1 cells

When Th1 activity is turned up,
Th2 activity is turned down
and vice versa

Th2 cells

Defense against
bacteria and viruses

Defense against worms
and other parasites

This is how children develop asthma, eczema, and allergies—their immune seesaw is out of balance and "stuck" with the Th2 police unit on constant high alert. But *how* does it get stuck that way?

During pregnancy, the mother's immune system changes to protect the growing embryo. It turns up the Th2 activity and turns off Th1, because Th1 cells would attack the embryo and lead to spontaneous abortion.[28, 29] As the baby grows, its immune system copies the mother's. Thus, the baby's immune system also starts out with the Th2 mode being active and Th1 switched off. From birth onwards, that gradually begins to change: As the baby's immune system encounters bacteria which stimulate its Th1 activity, the Th2 immune response is turned down. The alarm is turned off, the police units take a well-deserved break, and the immune seesaw is balanced.

This is where things go awry for babies that end up with atopic diseases. We're much cleaner today than we were in the past. We bathe much more often, we use antibacterial soaps, we eat processed foods, we don't spend as much time in nature or around animals—so our environment contains much fewer bacteria than that of our parents or grandparents just a few decades ago. As a result, many more babies miss out on the bacteria that stimulate the Th1 activity which, in turn, switches off the Th2 activity. Their immune system remains stuck on high alert in Th2 mode and becomes hypersensitive to objects that enter the body via the lungs, the skin, or the digestive system—like pollen, animal dander, or certain foods.[26]

This explanation—the lack of bacterial stimulation causing atopic diseases—has become known as the hygiene hypothesis. The hygiene hypothesis is frequently misunderstood: It doesn't say that exposing our kids to colds and flus builds the immune system. It says that our immune system requires exposure to bacteria, and not just any bacteria, but the right kind of bacteria—friendly ones that our immune system has co-evolved with. In chapter 2, it's time to dive in deeper. Understanding how bacteria help to program our immune system is key to understanding human health.

THE MICROBIOME: HOW GUT BACTERIA SHAPE YOUR BABY'S HEALTH

You have some 40 trillion bacteria living in and on your body. They're on your skin and in your intestines, your mouth, and your genitals—they're everywhere. You even emit your personal microbial signature like an "aura," to the point where researchers can distinguish which people have been in a room based on the bacteria in the surrounding air.[30] In all, you carry around between two to six pounds of bacteria of more than 10,000 different species, and they outnumber your own body's cells by about 10 trillion.[b] Collectively, these bacteria are called your microbiome.

The human genome has around 22,000 genes, but our micro-

---

b   Researchers used to think that bacteria outnumber human cells by 10 to 1. New research
    is showing that the ratio is closer to 1.3 to 1.[31] Not that it really matters: the key takeaway is
    that you are the host of many, many bacteria, and they play a central role in your health.

biome has around 8 million—that's 360 times more bacterial genes than human genes.[32]

In fact, we've come to understand that our own genes alone aren't sufficient to carry out all our bodily functions.[33] Instead, a significant part of how the human body functions is determined by bacterial genes. These bacterial genes work for us as if they were our own. They enable our gut bacteria to help us break down foods, make nutrients available to us, and produce beneficial vitamins and anti-inflammatory compounds our bodies can't produce themselves. Our microbiome is involved in almost every aspect of our health, from acne and dental cavities to diabetes, obesity, ulcers, and cancer, to psychological states like anxiety and depression—as well as allergies, asthma, and eczema.[34] Perhaps this is less surprising if you know that 70 percent of all of our immune cells live in the gut, where they interact with, and are regulated by, our gut microbiome.[35] That's why immunologists describe gut bacteria as "a buffer and interpreter of our environment."[33]

To understand how gut bacteria influence our health from conception onwards, let's take a look at how the microbiome starts to develop in babies. Around 1900, French paediatrician Henry Tissier was one of the first to study the microbiome of newborn babies. He thought that the womb was sterile and that babies get their first dose of bacteria from their mother's birth canal during delivery and later through breast milk. Only in the past few years did researchers discover that healthy wombs *do* contain a small but measurable amount of bacteria: in the placenta, in the amniotic fluid, in the umbilical cord, in the developing foetus itself, and in the first poo (meconium) of newborns![36] The bacteria travel from the mother's mouth and intestines to the womb via the bloodstream, and likely also upwards from the vagina.[c] This is completely normal and nothing to worry about. For the growing baby, this is the first contact with beneficial microbes even before birth.

Tissier, however, was right in that birth is a key event for the developing microbiome. During birth, the baby is colonised by beneficial bacteria picked up while passing through the birth canal. For the first few weeks of life, the baby's microbiome closely resembles the mother's vaginal and skin microbiome.[d] When a baby is born by C-section, the bacteria it encounters aren't primarily the mother's but those of the operating room environment and medical staff. C-section babies have significantly fewer of a group of beneficial bacterial families called *Bifidobacteria*.[37] We'll return to the health implications of C-sections in chapter 10 of this book.

For the next three years, babies pass through a critical window for the development of their microbiome. The first one hundred days in particular are key to creating a healthy, diverse microbial ecosystem that prevents chronic disease. If this ecosystem tilts out of balance—a state called "dysbiosis"—the child's likelihood of developing inflammatory chronic diseases later in life increases.[37,38]

---

c   This could explain why pathogenic (disease-causing) bacterial infections in the mouth (like periodontitis/gingivitis) and in the vagina (like bacterial vaginosis) are both linked to preterm births—the body's immune system launches a Th1-mode inflammation to kick out the bacterial invaders, and the foetus gets caught in the crossfire.[33]

d   Unfortunately, in many cultures, women are made to feel that their vagina is unclean or somehow "icky." Some women may cringe at the thought of having vaginal bacteria, let alone at those being a good thing for their baby. Yet, that's exactly what they are: they are natural, they're not unclean, and they play a really important role in protecting both the mother's and the baby's health.

In breastfed babies, *Bifidobacteria* and *Lactobacilli*—another beneficial type of bacteria you'll encounter frequently in this book—become the dominant species in the gut during the first few months of life. They are contained in and thrive on breast milk, which contains between 1,000 to 10,000 live bacteria from 700 different species per millilitre.[39,40] In this way, breastfeeding becomes the main driver of the baby's microbiome development in the first year of life.[41]

Lactic acid bacteria like *Bifidobacteria* and *Lactobacilli* help the baby fend off harmful microbes. By fermenting lactose and other sugars to lactic acid, they make the gut environment more acidic,[42] which makes it harder for bad bacteria to survive. They also produce natural antibiotics (antimicrobial peptides) which kill harmful bacteria while leaving the good ones unharmed.[43] At the same time, both *Bifidobacteria* and *Lactobacilli* stimulate the baby's Th1 immune response and turn down the Th2 response, thus lowering the risk of allergies.[44]

The interior of the gut has an enormous surface area to enable it to absorb nutrients. If you live in a city with sky-high rents like London, New York, or San Francisco, chances are your gut bacteria have more living space than you do: roughly 32 square meters or 344 square feet,[45] the size of a decent studio apartment. This also makes your gut an ideal portal for invading germs. But both *Lactobacilli* and *Bifidobacteria* act like your guard dogs. They strengthen the gut wall by triggering the growth of new epithelial cells which line the walls of the gut, thus making it harder for invaders to get through into your bloodstream. Additionally, they stimulate the production of mucus which adds another barrier to the lining of the gut, feeds beneficial microbes, and stops pathogenic strains of bacteria like *Esche-*

richia coli (commonly known as *E. coli*)ᵉ from clinging to the lining of the gut.

So what's the role of a healthy gut lining in preventing asthma, eczema, and allergies? When the gut lining is damaged and porous, tiny undigested bits of food, harmful bacteria, and other toxins can leak into the bloodstream. This so-called leaky gut causes chronic inflammation and allergy symptoms because the immune system begins to fight the invaders.

Bifidobacteria have even more tricks up their sleeves. Researchers have observed that they stimulate the growth of the thymus gland—the police academy in the baby's chest where Th1 and Th2 immune cells receive their "training." The thymus plays a central role in preventing autoimmune diseases in which the immune system mistakenly attacks the body's own tissues. Thymus function is directly related to its size: generally speaking, a bigger thymus is better.

At four months of age, breastfed babies have a thymus that is, on average, twice as large as that of formula-fed babies—roughly the size of a fig versus a grape.[47] Italian researchers wanted to find out whether they could increase the thymus size of formula-fed babies by enriching formula with beneficial bacteria and their fermentation by-products. In their experiment, thirty babies were breastfed, thirty babies were given standard formula, and thirty babies received formula that had been fermented with *Bifidobacteria* and another beneficial microbe, *Streptococcus thermophilus*. After four months, the thymus glands of babies who had received

---

e   Some strains of *E. coli* are a normal part of the healthy human microbiome and even help to defend the gut against invaders. Other strains of *E. coli*, however, are pathogenic and cause acute intestinal infections as well as chronic diseases.[46]

fermented formula resembled those of breastfed babies—larger and healthier than those of babies fed with standard formula.[48]

Bifidobacteria play yet another role in allergy prevention by interacting directly with the mast cells in the gut. Mast cells are a central player in allergic reactions. They respond to the presence of allergens by releasing histamine, which then triggers allergy symptoms like swelling, sneezing, itching, and wheezing. A particular strain of *Bifidobacteria* called *B. longum* docks onto mast cells in the gut and triggers their cellular suicide program (so-called apoptosis). This dramatically reduces the number of mast cells in the gut, which lowers or stops the allergic reaction to foods.[49] The amazing thing is that *Bifidobacteria* do this without weakening the immune response to real threats. Other immune cells that fight invaders (T-cells) remain unharmed.

The next major shift in the baby's gut microbiome happens when you start feeding solids. This introduces a much wider variety of dietary fibres. Fibres are carbohydrates from plants which our bodies can't digest on their own, but which are a food source for the microbes in our guts. After weaning, the ratio of *Bifidobacteria* and *Lactobacilli* decreases, and other bacterial species begin to colonise the gut. Your baby's diet determines which types of species grow most rapidly. In babies fed lots of meat and animal fats (common in our Western diet), *Bacteroides* and *Clostridia* become dominant, whereas in babies fed carb- and fibre-rich diets (common in developing countries), *Prevotella* becomes the largest group.[49,50] While *Bacteroides*, *Clostridia*, and *Prevotella* are all part of a normal gut microbiome, there can be problems when one group becomes overly dominant. You could think of it like a democracy: it's fine to have the largest party assume the role of government, but you need the opposition to keep them in check. Once you let things slide into a one-party dictatorship, bad things happen.

Around two to three years of age, your baby's gut microbiome stabilises and starts to resemble an adult one. When the microbiome is healthy and balanced, your baby's gut bacteria fulfil a range of important duties as part of their regular day job. One of them is the production of short-chain fatty acids (SCFAs). When it comes to SCFAs, the bacteria's trash is our treasure: SCFAs are the waste product of gut bacteria munching and fermenting dietary fibre. The most abundant SCFAs are acetate, propionate, and butyrate—and all of them are highly anti-inflammatory. Butyrate is the main source of energy for the cells in our colon, where it has been found to kill cancer cells and prevent tumour growth. Acetate and propionate provide energy to the liver, the kidney, the heart, and other muscles. Together, they supply roughly 10 percent of the energy our bodies burn.[51] Without butyrate, our colon cells undergo autophagy—that is, they literally eat themselves.[52] Butyrate is also, in case you want to know, what gives vomit its distinctive smell. That's right—our bodies are fuelled by bacterial waste that smells like vomit and protects us from colon cancer. The wonders of biology!

SCFAs like butyrate and propionate also kill bad bacteria that try to invade our guts, while leaving beneficial bacteria unharmed. Butyrate, for example, is used to treat acute *Salmonella* infections. Propionate is added to food as an antimicrobial agent. Both of these SCFAs stimulate the production of gut mucus and strengthen the gut wall—so much so that they are prescribed as medication or dietary supplements to treat the leaky-gut syndrome which is so often associated with allergic and autoimmune disease.[53] And it turns out that kids with allergies have significantly lower levels of butyrate and propionate in their guts than non-allergic kids.[54]

MICROBES, MOODS, AND BRAIN DEVELOPMENT

The effects of the microbiome extend way above your baby's belly. One of the hottest topics in neuroscience right now is the influence of gut microbes on our moods, behaviour, and even brain development and personality. According to John Cryan, a leading neuroscientist at the University College Cork in Ireland: "If you look at the hard neuroscience that has emerged in the last year alone, all the fundamental processes that neuroscientists spend their lives working on are now all shown to be regulated by microbes."[55]

In your baby's belly, in the lining of the gut, there is another nervous system—the enteric nervous system (ENS). The ENS is often overlooked but so extensive that scientists have nick-named it our "second brain." It stretches nine metres from the oesophagus to the bum, has an estimated 500 million neurons (five times as many as the brain of a rat), and connects to the brain through the vagus nerve and spinal cord. Scientists used to think that the brain was sending signals to the ENS to coordinate our digestion. Hence, they were shocked to discover that 90 percent of the signals passing through the vagus nerve were being sent from the ENS to the brain, not the other way around![56]

You'll know from your own experience that the "gut feelings" the ENS sends to our brain can have an enormous effect on our moods and well-being—think of "butterflies," the "sinking feeling" in your stomach, or simply the bad egg sandwich from this morning. In fact, even "artificial gut feelings" can produce that effect. In a small British study, eleven patients suffering from chronic depression which hadn't responded to any other treatments were implanted a small, pacemaker-like device to electrically stimulate the vagus nerve. More than half improved significantly, and three of the eleven patients were free of depression symptoms after a year.[57,f]

The neurons in the ENS and in our brain communicate using tiny chemical messenger molecules called neurotransmitters. You have surely heard some of their names before, because many of them also act as hormones in your body:

- Adrenaline/epinephrine, which jolts you into "fight or flight" mode.
- Melatonin, which makes you feel sleepy.
- Oxytocin, which gets you to bond with others and feel cuddly.
- Serotonin, which makes you feel happy and content.
- Dopamine, which gives you a sensation of pleasure and reward (many drugs work by activating the dopamine system).
- Gamma-Aminobutyric acid, more commonly known as "GABA," which gives you that "aaaaah" sense of relaxation (alcohol works by mimicking GABA in the brain).

And this is how our gut bacteria interact with our "second brain": They produce many of these neurotransmitters or stimulate their production in our gut. For example, our good friends *Bifidobacteria* and *Lactobacilli* produce GABA. That would

---

f   However, several patients in the study experienced severe side effects, like vocal cord paralysis lasting for months. Fortunately, if you are looking for ways to stimulate the vagus nerve, there are much safer and more natural options: aerobic exercise, deep breathing, meditation, yoga, tai chi, or cold exposure.

explain why breast milk, which helps these bacteria thrive and release lots of GABA, turns babies into "boobaholics"! Other species of bacteria have been found to produce serotonin, dopamine, noradrenalin—which also acts as an antidepressant—or acetylcholine, which is important for memory and learning.[58]

In a fascinating experiment at University of California, Los Angeles's Medical School, a group of healthy women ate two small cups of yoghurt daily, for four weeks. The yoghurt was enriched with "probiotics" (live beneficial bacteria)—*Bifidobacteria*, *Lactobacilli*, and two other species, in total about 28 billion living microbes per day. Before and after the study, the participants were shown a series of photos of angry and fearful faces, designed to trigger a stress reaction. Brain scans revealed that the women who had eaten the probiotic yoghurt had changed connections in some parts of their brain (again, after just four weeks!), which led them to react much more calmly to the stressful images than the placebo group who hadn't received probiotics.[59] Yet more studies have discovered similar results. In one, taking a daily probiotic supplements of 3 billion units *Lactobacillus helveticus* and *Bifidobacterium longum* for a month led to lower levels of anxiety, anger, hostility, and physical stress symptoms as well as better problem-solving in healthy volunteers. In another, 6.5 billion units of *Lactobacillus casei* per day for three weeks improved moods in people who were initially depressed.[60-63]

Feeding your beneficial bacteria achieves similar results. The term for fibres which our bodies can't break down on their own but which provide fuel to beneficial gut bacteria is *prebiotics* (as opposed to probiotics, the live bacteria themselves). One such prebiotic has the somewhat unwieldy name galacto-oligosaccharides (GOS). GOS is the substance in breast milk that helps *Bifidobacteria* and *Lactobacilli* thrive. In an experiment at the University of Oxford, healthy adult volunteers were given just 5.5 grams, about a teaspoon, of GOS per day for three weeks. The effect was similar to taking antidepressants. The prebiotic group scored lower on measures of anxiety and depression than the placebo group, and they also had lower levels of the stress hormone cortisol.[64,65] What's important to know is that these types of prebiotic fibres are not just in breast milk—they are a major component of plant-based foods.

As you can see, our gut bacteria have an enormous influence not just on our physical health, but also our mental health. Changing your diet will literally change your and your baby's brain. We'll return to the relationship between diet, the microbiome, and health in more detail in chapters 4–7, where we discuss which foods and supplements are most beneficial during pregnancy.

HOW TO CHANGE YOUR BABY'S GENES THROUGH EPIGENETICS

You may think of your genes as something that is set in stone when you're born, and you have either won the "genetic lottery" or you haven't. But we now know that this isn't entirely true—only to a certain degree. Your genes may give you a better chance of good health or a higher risk for certain illnesses, but those outcomes aren't fixed. Your odds for health or illness are fluctuating constantly during your lifetime because the activity of your genes is changed by your diet and lifestyle, and *those changes can be inherited by your kids.* This process is called epigenetics—the *expression* of genes. Epigenetics influence your children's health, and possibly even your grandchildren's, long before they are born.

So how does this work? To begin with, each of the 37 trillion cells in your body starts out with exactly the same DNA and genes. But if they're genetically all the same, how does a cell know whether to become a part of your eye, a part of your gut, or a part of your skin? How does it know how to do its job once it has become an eye cell, gut cell, or skin cell?

Imagine each cell as a little factory. These factories are pumping out proteins which do all the essential work in our bodies—like fighting infections, breaking down foods, transporting oxygen, making muscles contract and move, or carrying messages to other cells in other organs. The factory itself is controlled by a bunch of software—your genes. Each gene is like a line of code in a tremendously complex software program. Together, these lines of genetic code make up your unique genome. Your genetic code is stored in tightly wound spirals, the famous double-helix strands of DNA.

Each new cell starts out with a complete copy of your DNA and genes, but not all genes are being activated at the same time—that would be a disaster, as the cell would grow out of control. Instead, different genes are switched on in different cells, determining what kind of cell it will become. For example, in cells that become part of your eyes, genes are turned on to produce proteins that respond to light.

But what switches the genes on or off? Primarily, this is done by other genes within your genome: Roughly 8 percent of your genes produce proteins (so-called transcription factors) that activate or silence other genes.[66] Since these transcription factors are permanently encoded in your genome, there isn't much you can do to change them—yet.[g] The other way that genes get turned on and off, and this is a relatively recent discovery, is external to your genome. Genes can be turned on and off by chemical compounds from our environment and lifestyle: food, medicines, pesticides, and everything else our bodies are exposed to. The sum of these chemical compounds is called the epigenome—literally meaning "above/upon the genome"— and the study of how these chemical compounds influence the expression of our genes is called epigenetics.[67]

There are two main mechanisms for turning genes on and off. They are called DNA methylation and histone modification. If you are curious about how they work, the "DNA Methylation and Histone Modification" box contains some more technical details—if not, feel free to skip right past it.

---

g   That might change in the future as gene therapy or genome editing become more common, especially using new technologies like CRISPR—a way to cut, copy, and paste genetic code into gene sequences with incredible precision.

DNA METHYLATION AND HISTONE MODIFICATION

There are two main ways in which chemical compounds activate or deactivate genes. The first is called DNA methylation and has been likened to an "on/off switch." In DNA methylation, a gene remains switched off, or methylated, as long as a small methyl molecule clings to the gene. This "off switch" acts like a marker on the gene that tells the cell to ignore this particular bit of genetic code. Once the methyl molecule is removed from the gene, the gene is "switched on," and its genetic code is used to control the activity of the cell. DNA methylation is a fairly stable epigenetic modification that can be inherited, and it can also be changed by diet and lifestyle over time. Here's a little sketch to illustrate DNA methylation:

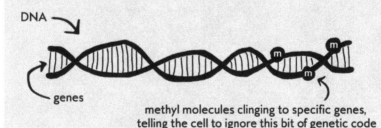

DNA

genes

methyl molecules clinging to specific genes, telling the cell to ignore this bit of genetic code

The second way in which chemical compounds activate or deactivate genes is called histone modification and has been likened to a "volume dial." Within our chromosomes, the strands of DNA are tightly coiled around proteins called histones. Imagine a string of beads: the DNA is like a string that ties the histone beads together and also wraps around them. Certain chemical compounds, so-called enzymes, can dock onto a histone bead and cause it to unravel the section of DNA that is coiled around it. Once that particular section of DNA is unravelled, the cell can access the genes. It reads the genetic code and begins to produce the corresponding proteins. The more unravelled the section of DNA, the more proteins are being produced–like a "volume dial." When the DNA is rolled back up into a tight coil around the histone, the genetic code becomes inaccessible and the gene is switched off. This "volume dial" is pretty flexible and reacts to short-term changes in your environment, e.g., stress or alcohol. Here is a sketch of how it works:

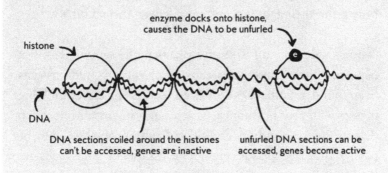

enzyme docks onto histone, causes the DNA to be unfurled

histone

DNA

DNA sections coiled around the histones can't be accessed, genes are inactive

unfurled DNA sections can be accessed, genes become active

Let's now talk about a specific example of how epigenetic modification can affect your health and, through inheritance, that of your children. Take BPA, the plastic compound often used in the lining of cans and, until recently, also in baby bottles and sippy cups. Researchers at the Duke University Medical Center studied the effect of BPA on a particular gene, the so-called agouti gene. All mammals have the agouti gene, and the mouse version is 85 percent identical to the human one.

In the experiments at Duke, healthy mice were fed foods laced with BPA. The BPA removed the DNA methylation markers from the agouti gene, thus switching it on. The babies of the BPA-fed mice inherited this switched-on agouti gene. As a result, they developed yellow fur (as opposed to the regular brown fur of their parents), became obese, prone to cancers and other diseases, and had a shorter lifespan. However, when the parent mice were fed *both* BPA and a methyl-rich diet (with essential nutrients like folic acid and choline), the gene remained methylated—thus switched off. The parent mice remained healthy, and their babies were born healthy as well.[68] Impressively, a methyl-rich diet was even able to *reverse* the damage: when obese yellow mice with switched-on agouti genes were fed a methyl-rich diet during pregnancy, their babies were born healthy and with brown fur, their agouti genes having been turned off.[69]

A quick side note on BPA and plastics: the same link—BPA exposure during pregnancy causing obesity in children—has been found in humans.[70] BPA is an "endocrine disruptor" that messes with your hormones, which can result in cancers, birth defects in your children, and other health problems. Unfortunately, "BPA-free" plastics are not necessarily better. It turns out that most of the plastics that have replaced BPA—and which are now used in baby bottles and sippy cups instead—are endocrine disruptors, too.[71] Therefore, it's better to go with glass or stainless steel whenever you can. For a look into the dirty politics behind BPA-free plastics, check out Mariah Blake's investigation, "The Scary New Evidence on BPA-Free Plastics."[72]

Another example of epigenetics at work: shockingly, more than 12 percent of pregnant women in the United States still smoke daily despite the many well-known health risks to their baby. When researchers analysed the DNA of their babies, they found that it resembled that of adult smokers—with genes switched on which are linked to smoking-related cancers, impaired lung and nervous system development, and birth defects like cleft lip and palate.[73]

Of course, fathers don't get a free pass for unhealthy habits. Smoking, junk food, or other chemical exposures leave epigenetic traces in their DNA which are passed on through their sperm.[74,75] The laws of epigenetics apply to fathers just as they do to mothers—and under some circumstances, even more so. A large meta-analysis investigated the parental alcohol consumption of nearly 42,000 babies born with congenital heart diseases.[76,77] The result was surprising. Overall, the father's alcohol consumption had a larger effect on the baby's congenital heart disease risk than did that of the mother's. When fathers engaged in binge drinking (defined as five or more drinks per sitting) in the three months before conception, their baby's risk of congenital heart defects increased by 52 percent, compared to fathers who didn't drink at all. When mothers did the binge drinking before conception, the baby's congenital heart disease risk increased by only 16 percent.

The good news is that, as we have seen in the example of the agouti mice above, epigenetic damage can be reversed with a healthier diet and lifestyle.

With this, let's return to the original topic of this chapter: the microbiome. What does the microbiome have to do with epigenetics? As it turns out, quite a lot. There is evidence that our gut bacteria are one of the *main drivers of epigenetic changes* in our DNA via the chemical substances they release in our guts—not just SCFAs and neurotransmitters but lots of other amino acids, proteins, enzymes, and vitamins.[78]

Remember that we talked about how SCFAs supply our body with energy, kill cancer cells, defend us against bad bacteria, and strengthen our gut wall? We can add one more thing to the list: SCFAs also regulate the activity of inflammatory genes both via DNA methylation and histone modification. In particular, SCFAs like butyrate, propionate, and acetate turn down the activity of genes linked to the development of allergies, inflammatory bowel disease, obesity, and cancers.[79-83]

So what is the key takeaway here? It's that your genes aren't set in stone—you can change your DNA through epigenetics. One of the main drivers of beneficial epigenetic changes is a *healthy and balanced* microbiome. Thus, the question becomes, **how do you acquire, maintain, and protect a healthy and balanced microbiome?** That's what we'll explore in the remainder of this chapter, as well as the coming ones.

WHAT THE HYGIENE HYPOTHESIS REALLY MEANS: YES TO GOOD BACTERIA, NO TO INFECTIOUS DISEASES

We're making our kids sick by keeping them too clean—that's the essence of the hygiene hypothesis. It's true, and it's also frequently misunderstood. Let's see if we can clear up the misunderstanding.

The hygiene hypothesis was first proposed in 1989 by David Strachan, a London-based doctor, who noticed a strange relation between hay fever and family size. The more siblings (especially older siblings) a child had, the lower the child's risk of hay fever. Strachan suggested that colds and flus transmitted by the older siblings could protect against allergies by "training" the immune system.[84] This was the accepted wisdom in medical research until about fifteen years ago—but it turned out to be wrong.

Researchers began to realise that exposure to colds and flus *couldn't* be essential to establishing a healthy immune system simply because the human immune system is much, much older than these infectious diseases! Most of the major infectious diseases plaguing us today only began to emerge within the past 11,000 years, following the rise of agriculture—a mere blink of an eye in our evolutionary timeline. Around 11,000 years ago, humans moved into ever denser urban communities, which allowed these infectious diseases to spread.[85]

Our immune system, however, started to develop about 2.6 *million* years ago in the Palaeolithic hunter-gatherer era and co-evolved with the microbes then present in the environment. This gave rise to the "old friends" hypothesis: our immune system requires the company of these "old friends"—the friendly bacteria with whom we have shared our environment since the dawn of time—to develop properly.[86]

Soon enough, the evidence for the old friends hypothesis began to mount. It was *not* exposure to infectious diseases (like colds, flus, measles, or gastrointestinal infections like *Salmonella*, *Campylobacter*, or *Norovirus*) that helped prevent allergies, but exposure to friendly bacteria like *Lactobacilli* and *Bifidobacteria*! As you saw in the previous chapters, these friendly bacteria regulate your baby's developing immune system and balance its Th1 versus Th2 immune response—and they help your baby to *fight* infectious diseases. Researchers were also able to show that the more older siblings a child has, the more diverse its microbiome[87]—thus explaining Strachan's original observation that more siblings mean fewer allergies.

Confusingly, researchers kept using the name "hygiene hypothesis" for this new explanation. This has caused some unfortunate misunderstandings of what the hygiene hypothesis actually means. From my own experience of talking to other parents, many of them believe that exposing their kids to colds and flus—or their kids being sick often—will "strengthen their immune system." Unfortunately, the opposite is true: the evidence is that exposure to flu viruses in particular raise a child's risk of developing asthma by making lung cells more prone to allergies.[88,89]

The same applies during your pregnancy: you should be *more* hygienic, not *less*, when it comes to avoiding infectious diseases. Foodborne pathogens like *Campylobacter*, *Listeria*, *E. coli*, *Salmonella*, *Norovirus*, and some *Clostridium* species are especially dangerous, as they can lead to stillbirth or spontaneous loss of your baby. You should completely avoid unpasteurised milk and cheeses, raw and undercooked eggs, shellfish, poultry, and meat (especially when it's ground meat like hamburgers). Also, be extra cautious with restaurant/deli counter salads (especially things like coleslaw), deli meats, and sushi. When I lived in France, I loved my Camembert unpasteurised and my *frites* swimming in fresh egg mayonnaise, but during pregnancy, I made sure that everything I ate was well-cooked. I was obsessed with hygiene and food security. I treated raw chicken as if it was radioactive: everything it touched had to be decontaminated immediately.

The key point here is, don't misinterpret the hygiene hypothesis. Exposing yourself or your kids to germs that can cause illness won't train or strengthen their immune system and can in fact do the opposite. Instead, what you want is exposure to the friendly microbes which steer our immune systems away from allergies and inflammation.[86] The challenge is that in our quest to avoid infectious diseases through better sanitation, cleaner water and cities, refrigeration, and food hygiene standards, we inadvertently also reduced our exposure to our "old friends." So where can we still find them? In nature!

DIRT AND BACTERIAL DIVERSITY

In our Western societies, we are spending roughly 70 percent of our time in our own homes and 90 percent in urban areas.[90] What we need to do, quite simply, is to get out more! Besides its beauty and stress-busting benefits, nature is also the place to meet our "old friends." One Finnish study discovered that the closer people live to farms or forests, the more diverse the composition of bacteria on their skin (mostly species that live on soil, plants, and pollen), and the less prone to allergies they are.[91]

This is what researchers have found all over the world: contact with farm animals, especially cows and their straw, during pregnancy or in the first few months of life reduces the risk of asthma, eczema, and other allergic diseases by nearly 40 percent. The more contact the better, but as little as three visits to a cowshed provided a measurable reduction in asthma risk.[92-94] The same goes for dogs and, to a lesser extent, cats. Being in frequent contact with these animals has repeatedly been shown to lower kids' risk of asthma and allergic diseases. Again, the contact with pets is most beneficial when the baby's immune system is booting up—in the womb and the first few months of life.[95] If you own a dog or cat while pregnant, your baby will be born with significantly lower levels of immunoglobulin E (IgE) in their blood—that's the antibody that clings to potential allergens and triggers the allergic response.[96] Of course, if you happen to be allergic to pets already, it's not a good idea to get one during pregnancy—you want to keep allergic inflammation (and any other kind of inflammation) in your body as low as possible during pregnancy.

What about inside your home? This is where you can dial the hygiene down a notch. The higher the bacterial diversity in your house dust, the lower your baby's risk of developing asthma and allergies.[97,98] In a study of inner-city babies in Baltimore, Boston, New York, and St. Louis, researchers found that babies who spent their first year of life in a household that had cockroaches or mice, which contributed to bacterial diversity, had a 25–30 percent reduced risk of developing asthma and allergies.[98] Another surprising study from Sweden showed that in homes where dishes were being washed by hand rather than by machine, thus leaving tiny traces of food on the plates which allowed bacteria to grow, kids had a 32–34 percent reduced risk of developing asthma, eczema, or dust/pollen allergy.[99] The same study discovered that regularly buying food from the local farm, which meant bringing farm dirt and mucky vegetables into the house, also reduced the kids' allergy risk by about 20 percent.

Now, I'm not suggesting that hiding dirty plates under your bed to attract mice and cockroaches is a reasonable allergy prevention measure. When I was pregnant, I spotted a mouse sneaking into our kitchen (we lived in Amsterdam at the time, and there's barely a house without mice in Amsterdam), and I freaked out! However, it's okay to relax about a bit of dirt in the house, especially if it's from food, farms, nature, and being outdoors. Relaxing also means to stop scrubbing your house with aggressive chemical cleaning products—those do more harm than good, as you'll see in chapter 9.

CHAPTER 3

ANTIBIOTICS: WHY, WHEN, AND HOW TO AVOID THEM

Antibiotics are overused and overprescribed in our society, which not only presents a threat to the health of your microbiome but to global public health.

The purpose of antibiotics is to kill bacteria. It would be an understatement to say that they *also* kill the good bacteria and not just the bad ones. In fact, they kill *more* of the good bacteria than the bad ones they are supposed to kill, since most antibiotics that are being prescribed are so-called broad-spectrum antibiotics. Broad-spectrum antibiotics can reduce the diversity of bacteria in your gut by 30 percent, that is, they wipe out thousands of beneficial species—and it can take years for your microbiome to recover.[100-102] For example, antibiotics given to mothers during C-section birth or to newborns significantly reduce the amount of beneficial *Bifidobacteria* in babies' guts.[100] Some groups of friendly bacteria can get eradicated completely and never return, while particularly dangerous ones like *Staphylococcus aureus* and *Clostridium difficile* are increasingly becoming antibiotic-resistant and take hold in the gut.[103] Antibiotic-resistant *C. difficile* infections kill 30,000 people every year in the United States alone![104]

The irony is that by killing the good bacteria that help to protect us against invaders, antibiotics are making us *more* susceptible to infections, not less. And as you may already have guessed, researchers have found clear evidence that antibiotic use during pregnancy or early childhood is strongly linked to the development of chronic diseases.

In a study of over 193,000 children from countries around the world, antibiotic use in the first year of life raised the risk of hay fever, dust allergy, eczema, and asthma by 40–50 percent.[105] Studies in the UK and Denmark involving more than 55,000 kids discovered similar increases in risk (between 17–98 percent for the various atopic diseases) when the mother received antibiotics during pregnancy.[106,107] In Germany, researchers found that the higher the dose of antibiotics and the earlier they are given, the bigger the risk of asthma: children who had received more than five courses of antibiotics were nearly three times more likely to develop asthma, and children who were given antibiotics between birth and six months of age had nearly *quadruple* the risk compared to children who had never received any.[108]

So how did we get to this point? Why is it that up to half of all women in Western countries are prescribed antibiotics during pregnancy, or that an astonishing 40 percent of kids' visits to the doctor end with antibiotics being prescribed, or that the average child receives ten to twenty courses of antibiotics before they have grown up, or that almost a third of antibiotic prescriptions in the United States are unnecessary?[103,109,110]

It's not just doctors handing out antibiotics far too easily—we, the patients, are to blame as well. Many patients and parents think that antibiotics are harmless and have no lasting effects, so they are quick to demand them, regardless of whether they would actually work. Doctors report that they are frequently pressured by their patients to prescribe antibiotics—especially when the patient/child has already missed work/school, and they're just not getting better fast enough. From the point of view of the doctor, according to Jeffrey Linder, a physician at Brigham and Women's Hospital in Boston, "you're confronted with somebody who has taken half a day off of work to come in. It's unsatisfying to say, 'You're going to be sick for a week or two.' It's much more satisfying to say, 'I have the magic pill that's going to make you better.'"[111] So instead of spending fifteen minutes trying to persuade someone that antibiotics won't cure them, or risking bad reviews on the internet for "refusing to help" the patient, doctors cave in and prescribe. The point I'm trying to make is, if your doctor isn't offering antibiotics, you certainly shouldn't ask for them.

The flipside of the coin is that when your doctor *is* offering you antibiotics, you should ask whether they are truly necessary and whether there are other options you could safely try first. Doctors sometimes prescribe antibiotics as a precautionary measure, especially when they're not sure of the correct diagnosis. For example, the symptoms of colds and bronchitis (which are usually caused by viruses and thus don't respond to antibiotic treatment) can look very similar to the much more serious pneumonia (usually caused by bacteria), so doctors prescribe antibiotics to be on the safe side.[111]

This is also what happened to me during pregnancy. During a third-trimester routine visit to the doctor, traces of protein were found in my urine. The doctor suspected a urinary tract infection (UTI) even though I didn't have any of the symptoms like pain or burning while peeing. He urged me to immediately take a course of antibiotics, because UTIs—including asymptomatic ones—can cause preterm labour. I really didn't want to take antibiotics, but as an anxious first-time mother, I didn't want to risk a preterm birth either, so I relented and took them. A week later, the lab tests came back negative—I didn't have an infection. Even though our daughter's health turned out fine, it haunts me that I didn't insist on waiting for the lab results and thus exposed her to antibiotics unnecessarily.

My experience of being pressured to take antibiotics during pregnancy is not uncommon. Most of the prescriptions during pregnancy are for treating Group B *Streptococcus* (GBS) infections, bacterial vaginosis, and UTIs, and often they're not necessary. Let's look at each of these and see what your options and alternatives are.

GROUP B *STREPTOCOCCUS*

GBS infections are usually harmless for the mother, and generally in healthy people, but they can be very dangerous for babies—they are the leading cause of sepsis (blood poisoning), pneumonia, and meningitis in newborns. In the United States, it is standard practice to test for it in week thirty-five to thirty-seven of pregnancy, and if the test comes back positive, the mother is given intravenous antibiotics during birth.[h]

---

h   So why aren't the tests done just before birth, instead of weeks in advance? The standard "culture" test in which the bacteria are cultured from a vaginal swab usually takes forty-eight hours—thus, the results might not be back fast enough if done too close to birth. Faster tests which take only one to two hours are now available but are not yet used routinely due to higher cost. Hopefully, that will change as costs come down.

Many European countries, like the Netherlands (where we lived during my pregnancy) and the UK, take a risk-based approach instead. Rather than testing routinely for GBS during pregnancy, they assess each woman's individual risk, then decide whether to prescribe antibiotics. The reason is that GBS infections during pregnancy are very common and not always problematic. Up to a third of women test positively during pregnancy, and these infections can come and go on their own in a matter of weeks—yet GBS infections in babies are extremely rare. So, to avoid unnecessary antibiotic use, antibiotics are only administered during birth if the mother exhibits one of these four risk factors:

1. Has previously had a baby that developed a GBS infection
2. Goes into labour at less than thirty-seven weeks
3. Has a fever during labour
4. Has had her water broken for more than eighteen hours

I ended up having none of these risk factors. With the risk-based approach, the rate of GBS infections in babies is slightly higher (1 in 2,000 babies, versus about 1 in 3,000 in the United States), but a large number of mothers and babies are spared unnecessary antibiotics.[112]

You might ask, "But if GBS is so dangerous, and the US approach of routine testing *does* reduce the risk of GBS infections, why not just use it?" Because it turns out that the antibiotics may do more harm than good. According to a study of 21,000 births in the United States, antibiotics indeed reduce your baby's risk of a GBS infection—but at the same time, by harming your baby's beneficial and protective gut bacteria, they *increase* the risk of infection with other Gram-negative antibiotic-resistant bacteria like *E. coli* and *K. pneumoniae*. In total, when using antibiotics, the overall rate of dangerous bacterial infections, sepsis, and infant deaths *stayed the same*[113]—and as you have seen, the baby now additionally faces an increased risk of asthma, allergies, and other chronic diseases due to having been exposed to antibiotics. The study's authors, a team of doctors at the Illinois Masonic Medical Center in Chicago, thus questioned whether the current clinical practice of trying to prevent GBS infections with antibiotics made sense at all—given that antibiotic resistance was on the rise and Gram-negative infections have an up-to-ten-times-higher infant mortality rate than GBS infections.

Ultimately, there seems to be no easy answer for this. If you have risk factors for giving your baby a GBS infection, you probably won't have a choice but to follow the clinical practice guidelines and take antibiotics. But if you don't have GBS risk factors, consult with your doctor on whether you can avoid the antibiotic drugs.

BACTERIAL VAGINOSIS

Bacterial vaginosis (BV) is another very common condition during pregnancy. It's caused by a simple bacterial imbalance. In a healthy vagina, *Lactobacillus* bacteria dominate, but during an episode of BV, other species increase by 100- to 1,000-fold to take over. The symptoms of BV are fishy-smelling white or grey vaginal discharge, and occasionally a burning sensation while peeing. Like Group B *Streptococcus*, it can resolve on its own, but because BV increases the risk of preterm births, the standard treatment is a course of oral or vaginal antibiotics. Between 20–50 percent of women in the United States and 5–15 percent in Western Europe are diagnosed with it during pregnancy.[114,115] Why the big difference between the United States and Western Europe? Because BV is often caused by vaginal douching and antibiotic use, both of which are more common in the United States.[116] Ironically, both douching and antibiotics are supposed to prevent or treat BV in the first place, but instead they can become the cause.

Let's quickly dispel some myths about douching and vaginal soaps. Most women who douche have been led to believe, by the marketing for vaginal cleansing products and by cultural norms, that douching is necessary to keep their vaginas clean, healthy, and non-smelly. The opposite is the case—because douching destroys your vaginal microbiome, it hasn't just been linked to BV but also to preterm births, ectopic pregnancies,[i] increased risk of sexually transmitted diseases (including HIV), endometriosis (an inflammation of the uterus caused by infection), and cervical cancer.[116–118] In short, don't douche—it causes serious damage.

Instead, it's best to let the vagina self-clean by restoring its natural balance of bacteria. This is also the best way of treating BV once you have it. At least three studies have compared the effectiveness of probiotics versus antibiotics in treating BV. The first found that vaginal capsules containing a small dose of only 10 million *Lactobacillus acidophilus* bacteria were just as effective as vaginal antibiotic capsules;[119] the second showed that vaginal capsules containing 2 billion viable *Lactobacillus rhamnosus* and *reuteri* bacteria had a 40 percent higher cure rate than antibiotic gel.[120] The third study used a daily oral probiotic containing 1 billion *Lactobacillus brevis, salivarus,* and *plantarum* bacteria instead of vaginal capsules. Eighteen women received the probiotic versus sixteen women who received a placebo. Within

---

i   In ectopic pregnancies, the foetus develops outside the womb and is not viable. Ectopic pregnancies are a leading cause of death for the mother because ruptures from the growing foetus cause internal bleeding.

seven days, the BV had cleared in all the women in the probiotic group, a cure rate of 100 percent versus a cure rate of 12 percent in the placebo group.[121]

You can also restore the balance of the vaginal microbiome by creating the conditions that let good bacteria flourish. *Lactobacillus* bacteria prefer acidic environments, whereas bad microbes struggle in those conditions. In one study, women received vaginal capsules of 250 mg ascorbic acid—yep, that's plain old vitamin C—to lower their vaginal pH value.[j] The result: after six days, 55–86 percent of women had been cleared of their BV, which is a higher cure rate than with standard antibiotic treatments. Both probiotic and vitamin treatments are available over the counter without a prescription, and they're cheaper than antibiotics—not to mention much safer.

So if your doctor wants to prescribe antibiotics for a case of BV during pregnancy, discuss if you can try one to two weeks of probiotic capsules and/or vitamin C tablets first. If you *must* use antibiotics, you may want to use probiotics alongside them—not only does it increase the cure rate, but it helps re-establish a healthy microbiome after the antibiotic treatment has ended.[122] We will come back to this topic at the end of the chapter.

URINARY TRACT INFECTIONS

UTIs affect about 8 percent of pregnant women. Often, UTIs are triggered by BV in which pathogenic bacteria travel up from the vagina and take hold in the bladder. The culprit in most cases is, once again, *E. coli* bacteria. If left untreated, UTIs can

---

j   The brand of tablets used in the trial is specifically designed for vaginal use and is called, imaginatively, Vagi C.

develop into dangerous kidney infections which may lead to premature birth. The symptoms include:

- Pain or burning while peeing.
- The need to pee much more than usual (though show me a pregnant woman who doesn't feel that way).
- Blood or mucus in your urine, or the urine looking cloudy.
- Urine smelling bad or unusually strong.
- Cramps, pain, or feeling of pressure in the lower abdomen/ bladder area.
- Pain during sex.
- Chills, fever, nausea, vomiting, back pain—these are indicators that the infection has spread to the kidneys.

Like BV, UTIs can occur without physical symptoms. The standard treatment, if diagnosed, is a course of antibiotics. Unfortunately, it seems that there is no easy way of getting around that—as far as I'm aware, there are no studies yet showing successful alternative treatments.

However, you can do things to *prevent* UTIs from occurring in the first place. In clinical trials with women who suffered from recurring UTIs, the women received vaginal probiotic capsules containing *Lactobacillus* bacteria. The trial participants used them daily for five days, and thereafter once a week for ten weeks. Over the duration of the clinical trial, the women showed a roughly 50–75 percent reduced risk of UTIs.[123,124] Numerous other studies have also confirmed the old folk wisdom that cranberry juice can help prevent UTIs: drinking a small glass daily of unsweetened cranberry juice (you can dilute it with water if it's too sour) reduces the risk by about 20 percent.[123] Cranberry juice does this by stopping bacteria from clinging to the inside of your bladder. I became addicted to cranberry juice during my pregnancy—I found the sourness refreshing, and it helped cut through the nausea in the first trimester. As a bonus, it exposes your baby's developing taste buds to sour flavours, making them a better eater later on (see also the section "Your Baby's Developing Taste Buds" in chapter 6). Another promising alternative being studied for UTI prevention is berberine, a plant extract that is both antimicrobial and prevents *E. coli* from sticking to the cells in your urinary tract. Unfortunately, unlike probiotics and cranberry juice, it's not safe during pregnancy.[123]

If you suspect you might be developing a UTI or your symptoms are still very mild, discuss with your doctor whether you can try vaginal probiotics and cranberry juice first.

ANTIBIOTICS DURING BREASTFEEDING

Antibiotics are prescribed just as frequently during breastfeeding as during pregnancy—in fact, they are the most common medication given to new mothers.[125] Like everything you consume, antibiotics are passed on to the baby through the breast milk. However, not all antibiotics are transferred through breast milk at the same rate, and not all are considered equally safe for the baby. So let's answer two questions. First, how do you avoid antibiotics during breastfeeding? Second, if you can't avoid them, how do you minimise the health effects on your baby?

The most common reasons for antibiotic prescriptions to new mothers are endometritis, surgical site infections, and mastitis. Let's look at each of these in turn.

Endometritis is an inflammation of the uterus lining, frequently due to a bacterial infection. It occurs in about 1–3 percent of mothers after vaginal delivery, 5–15 percent of mothers after a planned C-section, and 20–35 percent of mothers after an unplanned C-section following long labour with ruptured membranes.[126] Symptoms include fever, lower abdominal pain, and abnormal vaginal bleeding or discharge. Endometritis is generally treated with a course of intravenous antibiotics.

Due to the rise in antibiotic resistance, researchers are now investigating probiotics as an alternative treatment option. Unfortunately, the only studies so far involve mice and dairy cows, which frequently suffer from endometritis. The results from these animal studies indicate that probiotics can reduce the inflammation and potentially also the risk of endometritis occurring in the first place, but they are not a viable replacement for antibiotics yet.[127–129] Given that the risk of endometritis is largely determined by the mode of birth, the best option for reducing the risk is to avoid a C-section delivery. We'll talk about this topic in detail in chapter 10.

Surgical site infections affect new mothers mostly as complications after C-section delivery in about 2–7 percent of cases. As with endometritis, there are currently no viable alternatives to antibiotic treatment[130]—and in any case, the mothers would have already received antibiotics as part of the C-section delivery. Hence, yet again, the best strategy is to avoid a C-section in the first place (see chapter 10).

If you are delivering your baby via C-section, whether planned or unplanned, there is one crucial thing you can do that will dramatically lower your risk of surgical site infections. Perhaps you already guessed what it is—taking probiotics. A team of researchers from Thailand, the United States, and Malaysia performed a meta-analysis of thirty-one different studies involving nearly 3,000 patients. The result: when patients took both probiotic bacteria and prebiotic fibre (the combination of both is called synbiotics) in the days following surgery, their risk of surgical site infections dropped by an astonishing 72 percent. Additionally, the synbiotics were effective in preventing two other common post-surgical complications: pneumonia cases also decreased by 72 percent, and sepsis (blood poisoning) cases fell by a staggering 91 percent.[131]

Mastitis is an inflammation of breast tissue caused by a bacterial infection. Mastitis is rather common—it affects up to a third of breastfeeding mothers.[132] The symptoms are breast pain, a burning sensation while breastfeeding, swelling, warmth, and redness. You might also feel ill and develop a fever. Mastitis is the leading cause of undesired weaning, i.e., mothers stopping breastfeeding before they had intended to.

Mastitis develops when breast milk is left stagnant in the breast either because of blocked milk ducts or because the breast isn't emptied completely during breastfeeding. Bacteria from your skin or your baby's mouth can enter the breast and start multiplying in the stagnant breast milk, which causes the infection.

The standard treatment is a course of oral or intravenous antibiotics. Even worse, the bacteria which cause mastitis, bugs from the *Staphylococcus* and *Streptococcus* family, are increasingly becoming antibiotic-resistant. Hence, probiotics are being trialled as an alternative treatment for mastitis, and the results are looking very good.

A study at the University of Madrid in Spain involved 352 women who were suffering from mastitis.[133] Two hundred fifty-one of the women were given a fairly moderate daily dose of probiotics (1 billion bacteria or "colony-forming units" [CFU]) for three weeks, either *Lactobacillus fermentum* or *Lactobacillus salivarius*. The remaining 101 women were given the standard antibiotic treatment. The result:

- After three weeks of treatment, only 28 percent of the women in the antibiotic group had recovered from the mastitis; 44 percent still reported some breastfeeding pain, and 26 percent were still in severe pain.
- In contrast, a whopping 86 percent of women in the probiotic group had recovered completely, and the remaining 14 percent reported only slight discomfort while breastfeeding. *None* had severe pain.

In an earlier, smaller study at the same university, ten women suffering from mastitis were given a daily dose of probiotics (10 billion *Lactobacillus salivarius* plus another 10 billion *Lactobacillus gasseri*). Within two weeks, *all* of them had completely recovered from their mastitis—there were no more symptoms, and any previously cracked skin in the nipple or areola had healed.[134]

Two other Spanish trials have tested whether probiotics can *prevent* mastitis. What's interesting is that even though the two trials were very different with respect to the participants' medical history and pregnancy stage,[k] they arrived at strikingly similar results: a daily dose of probiotics reduced the women's risk of developing mastitis by more than half.[135,136]

So far, so good, but what should you do if you *have to* take antibiotics during breastfeeding? Make sure to discuss the choice of antibiotics with your doctor and weigh the benefits and risks. According to a review by Dr Joseph Mathew published in the *Postgraduate Medical Journal*, the strategy for minimizing the effects of antibiotics on your baby should be as follows:[137]

- Choose antibiotics that have poor oral bioavailability. Even when these are transferred through breast milk, they are less likely to enter your baby's bloodstream (however, they would still affect your baby's gut microbiome).
- Where possible, choose topical (applied externally to the infected area) or local antibiotics.
- In some cases, it might also be possible to choose antibiotics which clear quickly from your blood plasma, and thus your breast milk.
- Stagger the schedule of breastfeeding and antibiotic doses in such a way that the baby is fed immediately *before* an antibiotic dose.
- At the time when the antibiotic concentration in your blood plasma/breast milk is highest, consider bottle-feeding instead where possible.
- If your baby is premature, discuss with your doctor whether

---

k   The first study included fifty-five women in the last trimester of pregnancy who had struggled with mastitis after a previous pregnancy. The study included only women who had *not* taken any probiotics or antibiotics in the last month. During the study, they received 1 billion *Lactobacillus salivarius* daily from week 30 of pregnancy until birth. The second study involved 291 women who had just given birth *and* who had just been given a dose of antibiotics during birth. These women received 3 billion *Lactobacillus fermentum* daily for the next sixteen weeks.

the standard antibiotic dosage needs to be altered to avoid drug accumulation and toxicity.

- Only if all of these measures fail, consider pausing to breast-feed as a last resort.

Dr Mathew's review includes this table of which antibiotics are generally considered "safe," "to be used with caution," and "not recommended" while breastfeeding:

"SAFE"	"EFFECTS NOT KNOWN/TO BE USED WITH CAUTION"	"NOT RECOMMENDED"
Aminoglycosides	Chloramphenicol	Metronidazole (single high dose)
Amoxicillin	Clindamycin	
Amoxicillin-clavulanate	Dapsone	Quinolones
Antitubercular drugs	Mandelic acid	
Cephalosporins	Metronidazole (low dose)	
Macrolides	Nalidixic acid	
Trimethoprim-sulphamethoxazole	Nitrofurantoin	
	Penicillins	
	Tetracyclines	

Make sure to monitor your baby closely for any effects that might be caused by the antibiotics—either non-specific (like lethargy, poor feeding, etc.) or specific side effects like diarrhoea—and consult your doctor if you observe any. In some cases, it might be necessary to measure the drug levels in your baby's blood and adjust the medication or breastfeeding routine.[137]

Dr Mathew's review also covers antiviral, antifungal, antimalarial, and anthelmintic (antiparasitic) drugs during breastfeeding, but these are beyond the scope of this book. If you are interested, you can find the review online by following the link in the references.

An obvious follow-up question is, if you are taking antibiotics during breastfeeding, should you (and perhaps also your baby) take probiotics to counter the effects of the antibiotics? Unless you are severely immunocompromised, the answer is yes. You'll find more details in the section "Should You Take Probiotics Alongside Antibiotics, and Are They Safe?" later in this chapter.

WHEN TO GIVE YOUR CHILD ANTIBIOTICS AND WHEN TO WAIT

When your little one is ill and in pain, of course you'd do anything to make them feel better as quickly as possible. You might be tempted—as many parents are—to ask your doctor for antibiotics as a "quick fix," and as discussed above, your doctor might be reluctant to refuse them even if they wouldn't benefit your child.

You can avoid giving your child unnecessary antibiotics by following these treatment guidelines for common childhood illnesses issued by the US Centers for Disease Control and Prevention and the Academy of Pediatrics, in consultation with your doctor:[109]

- **Sore throat:** Antibiotics should *only* be given if there is a positive test for Strep or another bacterial infection. The test result needs to be based on a rapid antigen test or a throat swab, not just diagnosed by looking in the mouth. Unless your baby is allergic to it, penicillin is recommended as a better choice than newer, broad-spectrum antibiotics.
- **Bronchitis:** Regardless of how long it lasts, bronchitis or other non-specific cough illnesses should generally *not* be treated with antibiotics. If the cough has lasted for more than ten days and specific bacteria are suspected, discuss with your doctor whether a round of antibiotics makes sense.

- **Colds:** Antibiotics should *not* be used to treat the common cold. The common cold is caused by a viral infection against which antibiotics are useless. Thick and even coloured snot is a normal part of the cold and *not* a reason for antibiotics unless it lasts longer than ten to fourteen days.
- **Sinus infections:** These should generally *not* be treated with antibiotics unless your child suffers from both heavy snot and coughing without any improvement for more than fourteen days. If there is improvement by day 10, don't give antibiotics, as they won't speed up recovery. If there are severe symptoms (facial swelling, pain, fever above 39.5°C/103°F), discuss an antibiotic treatment with your doctor, and if necessary, use the most narrow-spectrum antibiotic possible.
- **Ear infections:** Here, you have to distinguish between "otitis media with effusion" (OME) and "acute otitis media" (AOM). Most ear infections are OME: fluid in the ear without signs of an acute middle ear infection. OME should *not* be treated with antibiotics unless they last longer than three months. AOM, on the other hand, is diagnosed by symptoms like pus behind the eardrum, eardrum pain, distinct redness of the eardrum, or discharge from the ear. Unless there are other complications, it's best to initially just give painkillers and observe for two to three days. If the symptoms don't improve or severe ones develop (severe pain or fever above 39°C/102.2°F), antibiotics can be prescribed.

I know it's hard to wait when you see your child in pain, but you need to resist the temptation to resort to antibiotics too early. Avoiding them when possible will benefit your child's health in the long run.

The good news is that yet again, studies have found that probiotics can prevent your kids from needing antibiotics in the first place. When kids regularly take probiotics containing *Lactobacilli* and *Bifidobacteria*, they require fewer antibiotic prescriptions and benefit from:

- A 60–75 percent reduced risk of colds, coughs, and fever. If your kids *do* catch them despite the probiotics, the illness lasts only half as long. In the study, conducted by Tongji University in Shanghai, children taking the probiotics (10 billion *Lactobacillus acidophilus* and *Bifidobacterium lactis* per day for six months) also missed 30 percent fewer child-care days due to illness.[138] Another study with a twenty-time lower dose of probiotics didn't find a reduced risk of colds, but even at this extremely low dose, colds lasted on average two days less and the symptoms were less severe.[139]
- A roughly 50 percent reduced risk of acute ear infections (AOM) and respiratory infections.[140] In this Finnish study, children received 10 billion *Lactobacillus rhamnosus* and *Bifidobacterium lactis* daily until the age of twelve months.
- A roughly 25 percent reduced risk of pneumonia and 20 percent reduced risk of dysentery.[141] In this study, performed in India, the kids were given 2.4 g of prebiotic oligosaccharide and 19 million *Bifidobacterium lactis* (an extremely low dose) per day for a year.

Eating yoghurt with probiotic live bacteria appears to be just as effective:

- In three separate experiments with American and Japanese adults, those who received a daily portion of yoghurt containing *Bifidobacterium lactis*, *Lactococcus lactis*, or *Lactobacillus bulgaricus* bacteria were about 50–75 percent less likely to catch a cold or flu during the experiment. When they did catch a cold or flu, their symptoms only lasted about half as long.[142–144]

- In a French study, kids aged twelve to forty-eight months received a daily dose of yoghurt containing *Streptococcus thermophilus, Lactobacillus bulgaricus,* and *Bifidobacterium lactis,* together with 1 g of inulin, a prebiotic fibre. Not only did the children miss fewer kindergarten days, but they also exhibited improved social functioning.[145]

The beneficial effects of probiotics—whether contained in fermented foods or supplements—never cease to amaze me. We'll discuss probiotic supplements and how to choose good ones in the "Probiotics" section of chapter 7.

SHOULD YOU TAKE PROBIOTICS ALONGSIDE ANTIBIOTICS, AND ARE THEY SAFE?

Since antibiotics wipe out your good bacteria along with the bad, it would seem to make sense to replenish and restore your good bacteria with probiotics. However, this strategy has recently been called into question by the research community as well as the media. According to some news reports, not only are probiotics *not* helpful in restoring your gut microbiome, but they can actually *harm* its recovery.[146] Is this true? Should you take probiotics alongside antibiotics, or should you avoid them? Let's weigh up the evidence.

The benefits of taking probiotics alongside antibiotics have been clearly established. Several large meta-analyses combined the data from nearly forty studies which involved more than 10,000 patients. This is what they found:

- A very common side effect of antibiotic treatment is diarrhoea. Taking probiotics alongside the antibiotic treatment reduces the risk of diarrhoea by about 60–70 percent.[147-149] The most effective probiotics appear to be *Lactobacillus rhamnosus*, with a dose of at least 5 billion viable bacteria (CFU) per day, and *Saccharomyces boulardii* (which is not a bacterium but a yeast which was first isolated from lychee and mangosteen fruit and which is closely related to baker's yeast).
- The leading cause of diarrhoea when you take antibiotics is infection with *Clostridium difficile*, and more than a quarter of these infections lead to hospitalisation within a week.[150] As we discussed earlier, *C. difficile* is also becoming increasingly resistant to antibiotics—and antibiotic-resistant *C. difficile* kills about 30,000 people per year in the United States alone.[104] Yet again, probiotics to the rescue: taking them alongside antibiotics lowers the risk of *C. difficile* infection by 60–70 percent.[151-153]
- Probiotics also reduce the occurrence of other common antibiotic side effects like stomach cramps, nausea, rashes, fever, soft stools, bloating and flatulence, and taste disturbance by about 20–30 percent.[147,151,153]
- According to one meta-analysis of twenty-four trials with 4,415 participants, not a single one of the participants reported any side effects that could be attributed to the probiotics.[147] Another meta-analysis found that in otherwise healthy people, trials have confirmed probiotics to be "harmless" with "side effects similar to a placebo."[154] However, in critically ill patients, probiotics *can* have dangerous side effects. When the immune system is severely weakened (e.g., by HIV, cancer, diabetes, malnutrition, or immunosuppressive drugs), probiotic bacteria can enter the bloodstream

and cause blood poisoning (sepsis), heart valve infection (endocarditis), liver abscess, and even death.[155]

So, on the positive side, the benefits of taking probiotics alongside an antibiotic treatment are clear: less diarrhoea, a lower risk of dangerous *C. difficile* infections, fewer overall side effects from the antibiotics, and unless you're immunocompromised, it's safe.

However, on the negative side, a number of recent news articles suggested that taking probiotics alongside antibiotics could actually be harmful.[146,156,157] What gives? These articles were all triggered by a single study, involving just twenty-one participants, performed by a team of researchers at the Weizmann Institute of Science in Israel.[158] This study suggested that probiotics would harm—rather than help—the recovery of your microbiome. Let's take a closer look.

In the study, the participants all received a seven-day course of antibiotics. After the antibiotic treatment, the participants were divided into three groups: seven participants were simply observed without further treatment ("wait and watch"), eight received a twice-daily probiotic capsule of 25 billion *Lactobacilli* and *Bifidobacteria* for four weeks, and six received "autologous faecal microbiome transplantation" (aFMT) (not for the faint of heart: this means they received an infusion of their own stool, taken from *before* the antibiotic treatment, into the colon— essentially receiving a copy of their original, pre-antibiotic microbiome). The study then monitored how quickly the participants' gut microbiome would return to the original state for each of these three treatments. The gut microbiome of the aFMT participants was the fastest to return to its original state, which isn't very surprising, since they were given a copy of their own original microbiome. The microbiome of the "wait and watch" participants was the second fastest to return to the original state, while the microbiome of the "antibiotic plus probiotic" patients was the slowest, because it now included some probiotic bacteria strains which were suppressing "native" gut bacteria from the *Clostridiales* group.

In summary, the study concluded that when your gut microbiome has been wiped out by antibiotics, receiving a copy of your own microbiome (via infusion of your own stool into your colon) returns your microbiome to the original state faster than by doing nothing or taking a probiotic which contains different bacteria. But contrary to the news coverage of the study, we don't know whether this is good or bad—the study says so itself! It's entirely possible that having your gut colonised by some additional *Lactobacilli* and *Bifidobacteria* strains could be good for you. Nonetheless, perhaps because the study's title used the phrase "Microbiome Reconstitution Is *Impaired* by Probiotics," the news reports described it as bad.

And it's not even clear that probiotics *actually* slow down the return of the original microbiome—four other studies involving a total of 155 people found the exact opposite! They concluded that taking probiotics and antibiotics together protects the original microbiome and also restores it faster:

- In a Harvard study with forty participants, taking probiotics (*Saccharomyces boulardii*, 500 mg twice daily) together with the antibiotic treatment protected the participants' microbiome and led to less pronounced changes, prevented overgrowth of *Escherichia* bacteria (of which *E. coli* is the most infamous one), and decreased diarrhoea.[159]
- In another study at California Polytechnic State University,

forty participants received antibiotics followed by either a placebo or a daily dose of 41 billion *Lactobacilli* and *Bifidobacteria* for twenty days. After the treatment ended, the gut microbiome of probiotic participants returned to its original state faster.[160]

- In Tanzania, sixty-five HIV-positive women with BV received antibiotics plus either a placebo or a fairly low dose of 2 billion *Lactobacillus rhamnosus* and *reuteri* daily. After fifteen weeks, 53 percent of women who took the probiotics had a normal vaginal microbiome, compared to 25 percent of women who took the placebo.[161]

- In a German study, researchers transplanted the microbiomes of ten healthy people into a computer-controlled artificial gut. Then they tested how these microbiomes were affected by taking probiotics (*Streptococcus thermophilus, Lactobacilli,* and *Bifidobacteria*) either *together* with the antibiotics or only *after* the antibiotic treatments had ended. They found that taking probiotics together protected the microbiome against destruction, whereas taking them after didn't offer the same protection.[162]

Thus, if you do take probiotics to counter the effect of antibiotics, timing matters. Taking the probiotics together with the antibiotics is better than waiting until the antibiotic treatment is finished.

Other research papers and media reports have speculated about "the "dark side" of probiotics, comparing them to "cuckoos" that might push your native microbiome out of the nest and take over your gut.[163-165] This seems like a largely theoretical concern. In practice, most studies have found that probiotics don't colonise the gut permanently. When people stop taking probiotic supplements, most of the probiotic bacterial strains become undetectable in their stool samples a short while later. Only a few strains manage to stick around. For example, a few months after ending the supplements, *Lactobacillus rhamnosus* is still found in 10 percent of people who took it; *Bifidobacterium longum* is still found in about 33 percent of people.[166]

Whether probiotics manage to colonise the gut is highly dependent on both the individual and the strain. In most people, their existing microbiome resists the colonisation.[167] This is true even in toddlers: in a Danish study, 201 children aged eight to fourteen months received a daily probiotic with *Lactobacillus rhamnosus* and *Bifidobacterium lactis* (1 billion each) for six months. Right after the probiotic treatment ended, *L. rhamnosus* was found to thrive in only 45 percent of the children, while *B. lactis* was found in 84 percent of the kids. Their overall microbiome structure or diversity had not been changed by the probiotic supplements, which led the authors to conclude that the long-term health benefits of probiotics must come from some mechanism other than permanent colonisation.[168]

Where does that leave us with the original question? If you are forced to take antibiotics, should you take probiotics as well? Weighing up the evidence, I would say that the benefits of doing so have been proven over and over again in practice, while the risks are largely theoretical—unless you are severely immunocompromised. So when your doctor or healthcare provider prescribes you antibiotics, talk to them about taking probiotics as well!

PART II

NUTRITION, SUPPLEMENTS, AND INFLAMMATION

CHAPTER 4

FEEDING YOUR GOOD BACTERIA

As we have seen, the microbiome is fundamental to our health. So I find it amazing how quickly we can alter it by changing our diet. In one Harvard study, healthy volunteers followed an animal-based diet (meat, eggs, and cheeses) or a plant-based diet (grains, legumes, fruits, and vegetables) for five days. Both diets significantly changed the composition of bacteria in the gut, but the animal-based diet did so to a much greater degree— towards a more inflammatory state. Bacteria associated with inflammatory bowel disease and liver cancer, like *Bilophila wadsworthia*, became more abundant and active.[169]

This also means that you can shift your microbiome to a healthier, more anti-inflammatory state in as little as five days! Which foods, then, are best for nourishing the beneficial bacteria in your gut? Primarily, foods that are rich in fibre.

DIETARY FIBRE

Dietary fibre is the part of plant-based foods that we can't digest ourselves but which feeds our microbiome—that is, fibre is a so-called prebiotic. In particular, fibre boosts the population of *Bifidobacteria* and *Lactobacilli*, but also other beneficial species.[170,171] Broadly speaking, there are two categories of fibre, and both are important for your health:

- Soluble fibre, which dissolves in water and is the main prebiotic for our gut bacteria. There are different types of soluble fibre, like inulin, pectin, or raffinose, which are contained in different foods in varying amounts. Beans, lentils, apples, blueberries, nuts, and oatmeal are all high in soluble fibre.
- Insoluble fibre, which doesn't dissolve in water, provides bulk and helps your bowel movements. It can also act as a prebiotic. Again, different foods contain different types of insoluble fibre, like cellulose, chitin, hemicellulose, and lignin. Legumes, carrots, cucumbers, tomatoes, brown rice, couscous, and other whole grains are good sources.[172]

Fibre is severely lacking from most people's diets. Only 3 percent of American adults eat the government-recommended amount of 25–30 g (about 1 oz) per day. On average, Americans consume only 15 g (0.5 oz) a day, while Western Europeans consume 23 g (0.8 oz).[173-175] Our ancestors, who thrived off a mostly plant-based diet, ate as much as 100 g (3.5 oz) per day![176]

In terms of overall fibre content, the US Department of Agriculture provides this ranking of food groups:[177]

FOOD GROUP	SERVING SIZE	FIBRE G/SERVING
Whole grains	0.5 cup	9.6
Cooked beans (legumes)	0.5 cup	8.0
Dark green vegetables	0.5 cup	6.4
Orange vegetables	0.5 cup	2.1
Starchy vegetables	0.5 cup	1.7
Mushrooms	0.5 cup	1.6
Fruit	0.5 cup	1.1
Other vegetables	0.5 cup	1.1
Meat	85 g (3 oz)	0.0

Eating a good variety of plant-based foods ensures that you get a broad range of nutrients and fibre, which increases the diversity of your microbiome—and thus also your baby's. Processed foods which advertise "added fibre" usually contain just one type of fibre, typically inulin, so your gut bacteria won't benefit from the same variety.[173] Food companies use "added fibre" as a marketing strategy to make processed foods appear healthy, even if they aren't. Unfortunately, junk food stays junk food—adding fibre doesn't magically make it good for you. As with other nutrients, it's preferable to get your fibre from fresh, unprocessed foods.

Having said that, certain types of added fibre (galacto-oligosaccharides and fructo-oligosaccharides) are effective in preventing atopic diseases when given to babies in the form of prebiotic supplements—especially when the baby is formula-fed. Clinical trials in Italy and the Ukraine found that babies who received prebiotic-enriched formula had around 50 percent less eczema, about 66 percent less asthma, and 72–85 percent fewer allergic food and skin reactions than babies who were fed regular formula.[178,179] Breastfeeding should nonetheless be the first choice; you can find more details in chapter 11.

As we saw in chapter 2, our gut bacteria transform fibre into short-chain fatty acids (SCFAs) which are highly anti-inflammatory. Several studies have found that mothers who ate a high-fibre diet during pregnancy had increased blood levels of the SCFA acetate[1] and decreased blood markers of inflammation.[181,182] This had profound effects on their babies' health. Their asthma risk was 50 percent lower, and the high-fibre diet had delivered positive epigenetic changes in the babies' lungs: genes that trigger allergic airway diseases had been suppressed.[181]

The easiest, and in my opinion the tastiest, way to consume lots of fibre is to follow the Mediterranean diet, which is inspired by the traditional eating habits of Greece, southern Italy, and Spain. It's like a beautiful summer holiday but on a plate. Fish, fresh vegetables and herbs, beans and other legumes, accompanied by crunchy whole grain bread to dunk in green, grassy, peppery olive oil, and perhaps some nuts and fruits for dessert.

The Mediterranean diet includes only small amounts of meat, dairy, and eggs. Eating like this doesn't just provide you with a good amount of fibre but also plenty of healthy fats and other important nutrients which are often deficient in pregnancy. The Mediterranean diet has well-documented effects on lowering your risk of heart disease, cancer, Parkinson's disease, and Alzheimer's disease[183]—and protecting your baby from asthma and

---

1   Interestingly, I came across a study which showed that drinking a tablespoon of apple cider vinegar per day also elevates acetate blood levels—which leads to significant weight loss, especially of visceral belly fat (the fat around your organs, which is the most dangerous for your health).[180]

allergies. A study in Spain tracked the health of 460 children, all living on the stunning Balearic island of Menorca, from before birth to six years of age. The children whose mothers adhered closely to the Mediterranean diet had a 40 percent lower risk of allergies and a roughly 70–75 percent lower chance of developing asthma.[184]

YOGHURT AND FERMENTED FOODS

Not a fan of Mediterranean cooking? An easy way to boost your microbiome and your levels of SCFAs is to eat yoghurt. The bacteria in your gut digest the yoghurt's lactose (the sugars naturally occurring in milk) into the SCFAs butyrate, propionate, and acetate. The yoghurt can be shop-bought or homemade, but make sure that it contains live probiotic bacteria. These probiotic bacteria—usually *Lactobacillus bulgaricus* and *Streptococcus thermophilus*—support the digestion of lactose and even alleviate lactose intolerance. This benefit is lost in heat-treated, pasteurised yoghurt.[185]

Moreover, there is strong evidence that feeding your toddler yoghurt is a great eczema and allergy prevention strategy. Three studies in Switzerland, Japan, and New Zealand found that children who regularly ate yoghurt in their first year of life had a 30–70 percent lower risk of eczema and a 40–85 percent reduced risk of allergies.[186–188] There was a dose-response relationship: eating more yoghurt resulted in stronger protection against eczema and allergies. The strongest protection was found when children consumed yoghurt more than once a week between the age of six to twelve months. As an added bonus, one study found that regular yoghurt consumption improved children's social functioning in kindergarten and preschool.[145] However, most "children's yoghurts" and fruit-flavoured yoghurts are laden with shocking amounts of sugar[189]—about two to three teaspoons per portion. Some brands manage to stuff nearly two tablespoons of sugar into a small cup of kid's yoghurt! Instead, it's better to choose natural, unsweetened yoghurt and throw in some fresh fruit, berries, and a drizzle of honey to make it more appealing to kids (but remember that honey is not suitable for children under twelve months).

Besides yoghurt, a great way of increasing the number of beneficial bacteria in your gut is to consume fermented vegetables like pickles, sauerkraut, and kimchi (the spicy Korean version of sauerkraut), and fermented drinks like kefir and kombucha. If you haven't tried them yet, you should! Fermented vegetables are crunchy, tangy, salty, and savoury, which makes them a great condiment with almost every meal, while the drinks are slightly sweet, tart, and fizzy like lemonade. Our daughter *loves* sauerkraut and kombucha.

Humans have used fermentation for thousands of years to preserve food and add texture and flavour. Fermented foods are teeming with dozens of different species of beneficial microbes—about a billion bacteria per gram or millilitre, which means about 15 billion per tablespoon.[190–194] Two or three tablespoons of fermented foods or drinks thus give you about the same probiotic dose as the highest-strength probiotic capsules available in your local health shop! However, unlike probiotic capsules, fermented foods also contain vitamins, minerals, enzymes, phytonutrients, and fibre.

We have started making kefir, kombucha, sauerkraut, and kimchi at home because it's so easy, and so much cheaper than buying them in the shop. There are plenty of helpful guides online and on YouTube, and I highly recommend the books *The*

Cultured Club by Dearbhla Reynolds and *The Art of Fermentation* by Sandor Katz—considered by many to be the bible of fermented foods (you can find these and other recommended books at **www.growhealthybabies.com/books**). If you do buy fermented foods in the shop, check that they are unpasteurised, or else they won't contain live beneficial bacteria.

Fibre and fermented foods are not the only dietary items that influence your microbiome and the level of inflammation in your body. Fats and sugars also play a crucial role, as you will see in the next two chapters.

CHAPTER 5

GOOD FATS, BAD FATS, AND HOW TO TELL THE DIFFERENCE

"Fat is bad for you, and eating fat will make you fat"—this is one of the worst and most harmful ideas in the history of nutrition science. Food marketing and official dietary guidelines, which are shaped and distorted by industry lobbying,[195,196] have repeated it since the 1960s, to the point where in many people's minds this is a basic, unshakable truth. Food companies are cashing in on it by pushing "low-fat" products which replace the fat—and the flavour it carries—with sugar, salt, and food additives. This demonisation of fat is, according to a group of UK doctors and clinical researchers, "perhaps the biggest mistake in modern medical history, resulting in devastating consequences for public health."[197]

Fats are essential to the functioning of your body. Your metabolism contains literally thousands of different kinds of fat, more than 600 in your blood alone, which are involved in energy and nutrient storage, growth, immune function, brain function, reproduction, and many others.[198] As you will discover in this chapter, eating fat won't make you fat—but too many carbs and sugars will. Eating certain fats can even help you *lose* weight.[199-202] Likewise, you will see that certain "good" fats are anti-inflammatory and lower your baby's chances of being diagnosed with asthma, eczema, allergies, and attention-deficit hyperactivity disorder (ADHD), while also being crucial to your baby's brain development, motor skills, and IQ. Other "bad" fats, however, are highly inflammatory and have been shown to *increase* your baby's odds of developing atopic diseases. Unfortunately, our average Western diet contains *twenty times* as much of the bad fats as the good ones![203] This is relatively easy to fix if you know the difference between good and bad fats, and what foods they're in.

Let's look at the most common dietary fats and their characteristics. Most dietary advice is based on increasing or decreasing your intake of these four categories of fats:

- Monounsaturated fats (MUFA)
- Polyunsaturated fats (PUFA)
- Saturated fats
- Trans fats

Unfortunately, as you will see in this chapter, these categories are not that useful. The reason is that nearly all of these categories contain both good and bad fats. For example, some types of PUFAs are good for you, some types are bad. For each type, it also matters what foods they come in. Omega-6 PUFAs on their own (like in vegetable oils) tend to be unhealthy, but some Omega-6 PUFAs come in packages that are extremely healthy (like walnuts, which are rich in antioxidants and nutrients).

To simplify these devilishly complex considerations at least a little, below is a handy "Good Fats/Bad Fats Cheat Sheet." This sheet takes into account both the healthiness of each category of fat as well as the food groups they're generally found in.

GOOD FATS/BAD FATS CHEAT SHEET

GOOD	OKAY IN MODERATION	BAD
Monounsaturated fats (MUFA):	**Monounsaturated fats (MUFA):**	**Monounsaturated fats (MUFA):**
Olive oil and olives	Canola/rapeseed oil (only cold-pressed organic!)	Canola/rapeseed oil (regular, heat-processed variety—contains trans fats!)
Avocados	Some nuts (pistachios, brazil nuts, and peanuts) and their oils	
Most nuts (macadamia, almonds, cashews, hazelnuts, and pecans) and their oils		**Omega-3 polyunsaturated fats (PUFA):**
High-oleic varieties of sunflower oil and safflower oil (only cold-pressed organic!)	**Omega-6 polyunsaturated fats (PUFA):**	While Omega-3 PUFA are healthy, avoid large predatory fish (shark, swordfish, bluefish, marlin, tilefish, king mackerel, and some tuna species) due to ocean pollution
Omega-3 polyunsaturated fats (PUFA):	Most vegetable oils (sunflower oil, safflower oil, soybean oil, corn oil, cottonseed oil, and grapeseed oil)	
Seafood and marine oils (fish, krill, and algae)	**Saturated fats:**	**Saturated fats:**
Flaxseed/linseed oil	Animal fats (tallow, lard, and duck fat) and red meat (beef, pork, and lamb; preferably grass-fed)	Palm oil
Omega-6 polyunsaturated fats (PUFA):		Processed meat (ham, bacon, salami, hot dogs, and sausages)
Walnuts and walnut oil	Eggs and poultry	**Artificial fats/trans fats:**
Sesame oil, sesame seeds, and tahini	Dairy (butter, milk, and cheese)	Trans fats
Saturated fats:	Coconut oil	Hydrogenated or partially hydrogenated oils; many margarine brands
Fermented dairy (yoghurt and kefir)		

Is there an even easier rule of thumb for which fats are healthy?

There is! As with fibre, following the Mediterranean diet is a good and very enjoyable way to ensure you eat healthy, anti-inflammatory fats. That's mostly how we eat. In our house, we use extra-virgin olive oil in almost all our dishes.[m] Besides lots of fresh vegetables and legumes, we eat avocados, nuts, seeds, yoghurt, and a good amount of oily fish. We have some chicken, eggs, and cheese every week, and we mostly avoid red/processed meat and vegetable oils. To find out why, let's go into more detail for each category of fat.

MONOUNSATURATED FATS (MUFA)

Like dietary fibre, MUFA provide a health boost for your gut bacteria. In a study conducted in Spain, obese mice with inflammatory microbiomes were fed a MUFA-rich diet. The MUFA restored a healthy microbiome in the mice by increasing the number of *Bifidobacteria*, as well as decreasing the number of *Clostridia* and other inflammatory microbes.[204] A different Spanish study fed mice the same amount of calories with either butter or extra-virgin olive oil. The butter-fed mice developed microbiomes resembling those of obese humans prone to diabetes and heart disease, while the olive oil-fed mice had gut bacteria resembling those of healthy, lean humans.[205] The antioxidants in extra-virgin olive oil have also been found to stimulate the growth of *Lactobacilli* while suppressing bad microbes like *E. coli, H. pylori, H. influenzae, Streptococcus,* and *Candida* yeasts.[206]

---

m Just be mindful of the "smoke point" of extra-virgin olive oil—it's around 190°C (374°F). Oils have different smoke points. At cooking temperatures above the smoke point, the oils start to burn and degrade. This destroys the oil's beneficial nutrients and creates harmful free radicals instead. For the occasional high-temperature wok frying, we use high-oleic sunflower oil (smoke point: 232°C/450°F) or unrefined avocado oil (smoke point: 249°C/480°F).

The Mediterranean diet is high in MUFA, due to the liberal use of olive oil. It also plainly contradicts the idea that "eating fat makes you fat." On the contrary: MUFA can help you *lose* weight! A review of a dozen weight-loss studies in which participants ate either a high-MUFA diet or a low-MUFA diet found that, on average, people on high-MUFA diets lost nearly 4.4 lbs (2 kg) more fat mass.[200] One particularly interesting Spanish experiment even pitted a "no calorie restriction" Mediterranean diet, in which overweight and obese participants could eat as much as they wanted and additionally received free bottles of MUFA-rich olive oil, against a low-fat diet. Guess who lost 46 percent more weight? The participants on the high-MUFA "eat all you want" Mediterranean diet—and I'm sure it was a lot more enjoyable, too.[199]

In addition to the benefits for your microbiome and your weight, MUFA also decrease the risk of heart disease[207,208] and, through suppressing cancer-related genes, lower your cancer risk.[209,210] Extra-virgin olive oil, in particular, is highly anti-inflammatory and protects your brain against ageing, Alzheimer's disease, Parkinson's disease, and more.[211–213] The reason for all this goodness is its rich antioxidant content, which gives good quality olive oils their peppery, grassy flavour. The stronger the flavour, the more antioxidants!

Avocados are another great source of MUFA, representing roughly 68 percent of their total fat content. They're one of our daughter's favourite foods and the first food she learned to eat with a spoon. From when she was eight or nine months old, she would polish off a whole avocado in one go and, her face smudged green, wave her spoon and demand more. Like olive oil, avocados are stuffed with antioxidants, while also containing large amounts of fibre, vitamins, and minerals. They can satisfy treat cravings, too. Just google "avocado banana chocolate mousse"!

Nuts, besides being loaded with vitamins, minerals, antioxidants, and fibre, are also a good source of MUFA. The highest amounts are found in macadamia nuts, cashews, hazelnuts, almonds, and pecans. Walnuts, however, mainly contain Omega-6 PUFA, which are inflammatory (we'll cover PUFA in the next section of this chapter). Nonetheless, walnuts are rich in many other healthy and anti-inflammatory nutrients, so there's no need to hold back on munching them. The only nuts I would suggest enjoying in moderation are brazil nuts, peanuts, and pistachios. They have a slightly less favourable fat profile than other nuts (with comparatively higher amounts of Omega-6 PUFA and palmitic acid) and, more importantly, are more frequently contaminated with aflatoxin, a cancer-causing substance produced by mould. Pistachios, in particular, are the greatest source of dietary exposure to aflatoxin.[214]

Lastly, what about other vegetable oils that are high in MUFA? There are specially bred "high-oleic" varieties of sunflower oil and safflower oil. These can be good for you as long as you choose cold-pressed organic ones, otherwise they tend to be heavily processed and made from genetically modified organism (GMO) plants sprayed with pesticides. Another vegetable oil that is often marketed as healthy is canola/rapeseed oil. Personally, I would only use cold-pressed organic varieties, and even those only in moderation, because canola/rapeseed oil contains erucic acid, which is damaging to the heart in high doses.[n] Canola/rapeseed oils that are *not* cold-pressed—which

---

n   That's why both the United States and the EU limit how much erucic acid can be in food-grade canola/rapeseed oil[215,216]—and it is supposedly safe at those limits. But why take the risk if there are other healthier and tastier options?

comprise the vast majority—are extracted using extreme heat and a toxic solvent called hexane. Trace amounts of hexane remain in the oil, and the heat treatment converts some of the oil into harmful trans fats. A study of regular canola oil sold in the United States found up to 4.2 percent of the total oil content to be trans fats—definitely not good for you![217]

POLYUNSATURATED FATS (PUFA): OMEGA-6 VERSUS OMEGA-3

There are two major types of PUFA, known as Omega-6 and Omega-3 fatty acids. Omega-6 is in vegetable oils like sunflower, safflower, soybean, corn, grapeseed, and cottonseed oil, while Omega-3 is in fish and shellfish.

Both are so-called essential fatty acids, meaning that both are necessary for our bodies to develop and function properly. Our bodies can't manufacture Omega-6 and Omega-3 themselves, so we have to get these fats from our diet. However, our Western diet contains too much Omega-6 and not enough Omega-3. This is where the problem starts: too much Omega-6 leads to inflammation, whereas Omega-3 is anti-inflammatory and crucial for our brains. Consumed during pregnancy, Omega-3 improves your baby's brain development and lowers its risk of asthma, eczema, and allergies. In this chapter, you'll see why.

Humans evolved on a diet which contained roughly equal amounts of Omega-6 and Omega-3. The Western diet, however, which uses cheap vegetable oils in almost every meal and processed food, has about twenty times as much Omega-6 as Omega-3.[203] In short, we went from a ratio of 1:1 to 20:1! In our diet, Omega-6 usually consists of linoleic acid. Our body converts linoleic acid to arachidonic acid (ARA), which is essential for brain, muscle, and liver development. So far, so good—then why is too much Omega-6 a problem?

The reason is that Omega-6 and Omega-3 compete to be metabolised and incorporated into your body.[203,218] If your diet is dominated by Omega-6, your body will be saturated with ARA, which can be inflammatory, especially if you already suffer from chronic inflammation. At the same time, ARA can block the uptake of Omega-3 and thereby its anti-inflammatory effects.[219] In other words, too much Omega-6 can make you deficient in Omega-3.

There is another reason why Omega-6 fatty acids can be inflammatory, and yet again it has to do with our microbiome. Western junk food diets rich in Omega-6 and saturated fats foster the growth of bacteria like *Clostridia*, *Proteobacteria*, and the *Enterobacteria* family (including *Salmonella* and *E. coli*), which cause gut inflammation, celiac disease, and other inflammatory bowel diseases.[220,221] As we have seen, gut inflammation can lead to food particles leaking from your gut into the bloodstream, triggering allergies. Omega-3 fatty acids have the opposite effect on the microbiome. They feed beneficial microbes like *Lactobacilli* and *Bifidobacteria* which are anti-inflammatory, strengthen the gut walls, and help prevent allergies and chronic diseases in children.[222]

According to some medical researchers, the Omega-6 to Omega-3 imbalance is one of the drivers of chronic diseases in the Western world. A team of scientists at the US National Institutes of Health compared the consumption of Omega-6 and Omega-3 fatty acids across thirty-eight different countries. What they found was striking: the higher the Omega-6 intake and the lower the Omega-3 intake as a percentage of total calories, the higher the country's rates of heart disease, stroke, depression—and even murder.[223] Murder? Yes: Omega-6 and Omega-3 have profound effects on our brain and behaviour. An experiment with prisoners demonstrated that supplementing their diets with Omega-3 fatty acids reduced violence and aggression, while a study tracking the rise in Omega-6 intake and homicides over thirty-nine years and five countries (Argentina, Australia, Canada, the UK, and the United States) found that they correlated almost perfectly.[224] Dr Joseph Hibbeln, head of nutritional neurosciences at the US National Institutes of Health and one of the world's leading experts on the role of dietary fats in human brain function, summed it up as follows: "The increases in world [Omega-6] consumption over the past century may be considered a very large uncontrolled experiment that may have contributed to increased societal burdens of aggression, depression, and cardiovascular mortality."[223]

If the dietary ratio of Omega-6 to Omega-3 can affect entire societies in this way, you won't be surprised to learn that it also affects your baby's health. Studies performed in Finland, Germany, Ireland, and Australia have all concluded that the higher the ratio of Omega-6 to Omega-3 in your pregnancy diet, or in your breast milk after birth, the higher your baby's risk of developing allergies, asthma, and eczema.[225-229]

What's a healthy ratio of Omega-6 to Omega-3, then? The anti-inflammatory effects of Omega-3 become noticeable and the symptoms of asthma sufferers improve when you eat no more than five times as much Omega-6 as Omega-3, meaning a ratio of no more than 5:1.[230,231] Ideally, you would strive to consume equal amounts of each, or a ratio of 1:1.

Now that we've established the importance of Omega-3 fatty acids, let's take a closer look at what they do and how to get them into your diet. The main types of Omega-3 are EPA (eicosapentaenoic acid), DHA (docosahexaenoic acid), and ALA (alpha-linolenic acid). EPA and DHA can only be found in marine sources like fish, krill, and algae. ALA is contained in some seed oils, like flax/linseed, hemp, pumpkin, rapeseed/canola, as well as walnuts. Of these three types of Omega-3 fatty acids, DHA is especially critical for the healthy growth and development of your baby. It's the main building block of the brain, cerebral cortex, retina, and skin.

Researchers used to believe that our bodies are able to convert ALA to EPA and DHA. Based on this, many vegetarians and vegans assumed they could simply replace seafood with nuts and seeds to cover their dietary Omega-3 needs. Unfortunately, it turns out that our bodies are pretty bad at this conversion—of the ALA you eat, at best only 5–10 percent is converted to EPA and 2–5 percent to DHA. In several studies of flaxseed/linseed and walnut oil, the conversion of ALA to DHA was *zero*![218,232] If you follow a vegetarian or vegan diet, this means that unfortunately you *cannot* get enough DHA to cover your growing baby's needs from nut or seed oils. However, there is a vegan alternative to fish or fish oil supplements. You can skip the middleman—or middle fish—and go straight to the source: fish get their DHA by eating krill which eat algae, and algae oil supplements are a good vegan source of DHA.[232]

So what do Omega-3 fatty acids and DHA do for your baby? For a start, they help to balance the developing immune system's Th1/Th2 response, which (as you saw in chapter 1) is out of balance and tilted towards Th2 in allergic kids.[233] Eight separate trials in Australia, Mexico, the UK, and Scandinavia supplemented pregnant women's diets with fish oil capsules or oily fish. Their children were 87 percent less likely to develop food allergies in the first year of life, had a 40 percent lower rate of eczema, and a 34 percent lower risk of being diagnosed with any allergies in the first three years of life.[234] In three Norwegian studies, babies who started to eat oily fish regularly before the age of one were 25 percent less likely to develop asthma and allergies[235] and a whopping 76 percent less likely to develop eczema.[236]

But DHA isn't just important for preventing chronic disease—it is the primary building block of your baby's brain. Specifically, DHA is crucial for forming connections in the brain: Like a fertiliser that encourages a plant's roots to grow, DHA encourages brain cells to branch out and search for other cells to connect to. And not only does DHA lead to more brain connections, it also makes these connections work better. As part of the myelin sheath and synaptic membrane, DHA insulates the brain's wiring and connection points. This increases the speed at which electrical and chemical signals can zip around the brain.[237–239] In short, DHA makes your baby's brain healthier, faster, and more interconnected. As a result, there are tons of studies demonstrating how DHA intake during pregnancy boosts children's cognitive development: better visual perception, hand-eye coordination, motor skills, attention, problem-solving skills, language development, and participation in conversation.[240,241]

DHA can also reverse the epigenetic damage caused by sugar consumption, as well as protect the brain from inflammation by lowering the expression of inflammatory genes.[237,242] Conversely, a lack of DHA during pregnancy leads to poorer brain development and a higher likelihood of ADHD.[241,243] Studies found that if mothers ate less than three servings of fish per week during pregnancy, their children had lower IQ scores and cognitive development compared to children whose mothers ate more than three servings of fish per week. If mothers didn't eat any fish at all during pregnancy, their children had five to ten points lower IQ scores at age three to four.[244,245]

OMEGA-3 FROM FISH: WHAT ABOUT THE POLLUTION OF THE OCEAN?

In general, the research shows that eating fish is great for your baby's health. Besides DHA, fish is also a rich source of vitamin D, selenium, and other nutrients. But before you rush out to buy some for dinner, there are certain things to consider. The pollution of our oceans means it's not safe to just eat any fish, or as much fish as you want. Fish are constantly exposed to toxic heavy metals like mercury, industrial chemicals like PCB, agricultural runoff of fertilisers and pesticides, and consumer waste like microplastics. These toxins accumulate in their bodies—both in wild fish and in farmed fish that are raised in pens in the ocean.[246] The vast majority of farmed fish products also suffer from the same problems as factory-farmed meat: routine antibiotic overuse, low quality of life for the animals, and cheap plant-based and animal waste feed—which shifts the balance of fatty acids in the fish from Omega-3 to Omega-6.

It sounds so bad that it almost makes you want to stop eating fish, right? Well, I spent my early childhood by the Irish seaside where my parents ran a seafood restaurant. I love fish and wouldn't want to give it up. If you stick to a few guidelines, you can ensure that the fish you eat is both healthy and sustainable. First, seek out sustainably caught (MSC-certified) wild fish rather than farmed fish. If you can only find farmed fish, choose certified organic or skip it.° Second, as a rule of thumb, smaller fish species are less polluted than larger ones. The reason is that, as smaller fish get gobbled up by progressively larger fish, the larger fish accumulate the toxins contained in their prey. This cycle repeats until the top predators are, metaphorically speaking, swimming Russian dolls of toxic waste. The concentration of mercury (and other toxins) is highest in large, long-lived species like tilefish, swordfish, shark, king mackerel, tuna, and marlin—the general advice is to avoid these completely as soon as you're planning to become pregnant. In smaller or short-lived oily fish, like Atlantic mackerel and herring, the toxin concentration is five to twenty times lower, and in anchovies, sardines, and wild salmon, there are twenty to one hundred times fewer toxins than in the large predators.[247]

One of the main environmental pollutants that accumulates in fish is mercury. Because of these mercury concerns, the dietary guidelines for pregnant women recommend eating no more than two to three servings of seafood per week.[248] Yet, there is new research showing that—as long as we avoid the large predators—the mercury in seafood is not as dangerous as previously believed. Two Norwegian and Brazilian studies found that selenium, an essential nutrient that is abundant in fish, can block the toxic effects of mercury in our body by binding to it before it gets absorbed.[249,250] In studies with rats, even high doses of mercury did not have toxic effects as long as the animals were given an even higher dose of selenium.[251] Almost all fish contain higher levels of selenium than mercury—except large predators like shark, swordfish, some tuna species, and bluefish.[252,253]

An American-British study published in the leading medical

---

o Though organic certification for fish is highly controversial—the standards differ hugely from country to country, and animal welfare is lower than in organic meat farming.

journal *The Lancet* investigated the seafood consumption of nearly 12,000 pregnant women. Because of environmental pollution concerns, US dietary guidelines state that pregnant women should limit their seafood intake to 340 g per week. However, the researchers found that the babies of mothers who ate *more* than 340 g per week were much healthier, with higher verbal IQ scores, better motor control, and improved social development. The researchers concluded that the dietary guidelines limiting seafood consumption during pregnancy could actually be harmful.[244,245]

For pregnant and breastfeeding women, most nutritional guidelines recommend a *minimum* amount of 200–250 mg DHA per day.[254] You can get this amount from two to three servings of seafood per week. If you want to maximise the health benefits for your baby, you should aim to consume *more* than the minimum recommended amount of 200–250 mg DHA per day. In the studies I describe in this chapter—the ones that found DHA promoting brain development, motor skills, intelligence, and lowering the risks for chronic diseases—mothers consumed between 400–1,000 mg per day during pregnancy.[255]

Depending on the species, oily fish has about 500–1,500 mg of Omega-3 fatty acids per serving, of which about two-thirds is DHA and one-third is EPA. Fish stocks are constantly changing due to overfishing and (in some cases) recovery, so it's best to always check for the MSC certification when buying fish. Currently, the best options for sustainable, wild-caught, high-DHA oily fish are:[256,257]

- Anchovies (Atlantic), ca. 900–1,300 mg DHA per 3.5 oz/ 100 g
- Herring (Atlantic), ca. 1,100–1,200 mg DHA per 3.5 oz/100 g

- Mackerel (Atlantic), ca. 700–900 mg DHA per 3.5 oz/100 g
- Salmon (Pacific), ca. 700–900 mg DHA per 3.5 oz/100 g
- Sardines (Atlantic), ca. 500 mg DHA per 3.5 oz/100 g

Personally, when I was pregnant, I ate more than two to three portions of oily fish and wild salmon per week. I also started taking about 900 mg DHA daily in high-quality fish oils as soon as I was planning to get pregnant—and I continued taking them as long as I was still breastfeeding our daughter. But even though fish oil capsules are a wonderful supplement, it appears that nothing beats the real thing: one study found that DHA from fish is absorbed at a nine times higher rate than from fish oil capsules.[258]

If you decide to take fish oil supplements, it's crucial to choose high-quality brands which are purified, independently tested for heavy metals, and from sustainable sources. The International Fish Oil Standards (IFOS) Program has data for all reputable brands on their website, and LabDoor provides fish oil rankings based on quality and value for money. For more information on fish oil, there's a great, in-depth buyers guide on health author Chris Kresser's website. You can find up-to-date links to these resources via **www.growhealthybabies.com/supplements**.

SATURATED FATS

Saturated fats in our diet come from four main sources:

- Dairy (milk, cheese, butter, and ghee)
- Meat and animal fats (lard, tallow, and duck fat)
- Eggs
- Tropical plant oils (palm oil and coconut oil)

The idea that saturated fats, especially dairy and animal fats, cause heart disease has become enshrined in medical teaching and government dietary guidelines. It's an interesting case study in how science can take a decades-long detour, simply due to a single man's flawed work, shrewd politics, and sheer aggressiveness.

As Nina Teicholz recounts in her book *The Big Fat Surprise*, the hypothesis that saturated fats cause heart disease was proposed by Ancel Keys, a pathologist at the University of Minnesota, in the 1950s.[259] For the next few decades, Keys went about confirming his hypothesis by "cherry-picking" his data, suppressing evidence to the contrary, and aggressively attacking anybody who dared to criticise his findings. He successfully lobbied for his views to be incorporated into the American Heart Association's first-ever dietary guidelines in 1961, and the US government's dietary guidelines in 1977. Keys's allies held top posts in government and public health bodies, so critics were denied research grants and key positions on expert panels.

It took five decades until a new generation of researchers dared to challenge Keys's dogma, and their work is showing that Keys and his colleagues were wrong. Recent meta-analyses combining the results of dozens of studies, involving hundreds of thousands of patients, have come to the conclusion that eating saturated fats does *not* raise mortality or the risks of heart disease, diabetes, and stroke.[260,261] Advocates of saturated fats, especially followers of the Paleo diet, correctly point out that animal fats like lard, tallow, or duck fat contain almost as much MUFA as saturated fat, and MUFA are generally healthy and anti-inflammatory. Additionally, eggs, meat, and dairy can be rich sources of proteins, vitamins, and minerals.

However, for optimum health during pregnancy, stuffing yourself with steak and milkshakes every night is decidedly not a good idea. Poultry and eggs are fine in moderation, but your—and thus your baby's—health is likely to benefit from eating less red meat (beef, pork, lamb, and goat) and avoiding processed meats altogether (bacon, ham, salami, hot dogs, etc.). The reason is that both red and processed meats are inflammatory and classed as carcinogenic by the World Health Organization: if you eat the average amount that meat eaters consume per day, which is around 3.5 oz/100 g of red meat (roughly half a steak) or 1.75 oz/50 g of processed meat (four strips of bacon, or one hot dog), your risk of colorectal cancer increases by 17–18 percent—meaning your absolute risk of developing this cancer during your lifetime goes up from 5 percent to 6 percent. That doesn't seem like a lot, but it adds up to 35,000–50,000 cancer deaths per year globally.[262-265] When you *do* choose to eat red meat, make sure to eat it with some high-fibre foods like whole grains, legumes, or dark green veg, because this reduces the formation of the cancer-causing compounds.[266,267]

And what about dairy? Analyses by the World Health Organization show that high dairy consumption doubles the risk of ovarian cancer,[268] raises the risk of prostate cancer by 30–150 percent,[269] and—after a breast cancer diagnosis—increases mortality by 50 percent.[270] Several studies have also linked it to a higher risk of premenopausal breast cancer, colon cancer, and lung cancer.[271] The reason is that dairy contains a powerful growth hormone called insulin-like growth factor 1 (IGF-1), which is identical to the IGF-1 in humans.

What IGF-1 does is to increase the growth and proliferation of cells, while stopping old or damaged cells from self-destructing— and that is what can lead to cancer.[272,273] However, it turns out that not all dairy products affect the amount of IGF-1 in your body. Drinking milk raises your IGF-1 levels, while fermented dairy products like yoghurt, kefir, or cheese don't—because fermentation removes about 80–90 percent of the IGF-1.[271,274,275] Also, there can be enormous differences between the IGF-1 levels of various milk brands, especially between organic and non-organic milk. How come? Well, some countries permit non-organic dairy farmers to use a genetically modified artificial growth hormone called recombinant bovine somatotropin (rBST; sometimes also called rBGH for "recombinant bovine growth hormone") to increase milk production. The milk of rBST-treated cows contains roughly twice the level of IGF-1 growth hormones as that of non-treated cows.[276] The use of rBST is banned in the EU, Canada, Australia, New Zealand, Japan, Israel, and Argentina—but allowed in the United States, Mexico, Brazil, India, Russia, South Korea, and many Latin American countries.

Even putting the cancer risk aside—when you eat a lot of meat and dairy, their saturated fats can tip your microbiome out of balance and lead to gut inflammation. How does this happen? Saturated fats are hard to break down, so our liver produces bile to help our gut digest the fat. Bile is rich in sulphur, which feeds certain kinds of inflammatory bacteria like *Bilophila wadsworthia*—and suppresses our anti-inflammatory friends *Lactobacilli* and *Bifidobacteria*.[277–279] *Bilophila wadsworthia* produces hydrogen sulphide, which inflames the gut wall and makes it more porous—the opposite of what *Lactobacilli* and *Bifidobacteria* do—so food particles can cross into the bloodstream and potentially cause allergic reactions. *B. wadsworthia* is almost undetectable in healthy guts, but features prominently in people suffering from inflammatory bowel disease and ulcerative colitis.[277,279,280]

Additionally, saturated fats can also inflame our gut directly, not just by altering our microbiome. One of the first lines of defence that our immune system uses against infections are molecules called toll-like receptors (TLRs). TLRs are like puzzle pieces designed to attach to invaders like bacteria, viruses, and fungi. If a puzzle piece fits, the immune system recognises what kind of threat it is dealing with and launches an attack. Unfortunately, two of the main types of saturated fats—palmitic and stearic acids—fit one of the TLR puzzle pieces (called TLR4) and thus get mistaken for bacterial invaders. In response, the immune system releases cytokines to fight the supposed threat. The result is inflammation and damage to the lining of the gut.[278,281,282] Palmitic acid, by the way, derives its name from palm oil, now the most widely consumed vegetable oil on earth. It's also one of the most inflammatory vegetable oils and linked to heart disease in developing countries[283-285]—on top of being an environmental disaster.[p]

Now, what about coconut oil? It's somewhat different from the other saturated fats. Unlike all other saturated fats, coconut oil is low in palmitic and stearic acid; instead, it mainly consists of lauric acid. While palmitic acid is inflammatory, lauric acid is anti-inflammatory.[285,288-290] That is why, even though both palm oil and coconut oil are saturated fats and would thus be considered interchangeable in government dietary guidelines, they can have exactly the opposite effect on health. In one animal study, rats that were fed palm oil developed heart disease, while rats that were fed *both* palm oil and coconut oil

---

p   Huge swathes of rainforest in Indonesia, Malaysia, and Africa are being cleared to make space for monoculture oil palm plantations—the equivalent of 300 football pitches *every hour*.[286] This makes palm oil one of the leading causes of deforestation, which in turn contributes to climate change, soil erosion and flooding, and habitat loss for endangered species like orangutans. The Center for International Forestry Research calls palm oil "undoubtedly an ecological disaster."[287]

didn't—the antioxidants in coconut oil apparently protected the rats' cardiovascular system from damage.[291] I'm not aware of any studies demonstrating conclusively that coconut oil *prevents* heart disease in humans, but there are numerous studies showing that it doesn't *cause* it, while also raising "good" (HDL) cholesterol,[292-295] which is associated with lowering the risk of heart disease.

ARTIFICIAL FATS AND TRANS FATS

The case against artificial fats, like partially hydrogenated fats or trans fats, is straightforward. They are among the worst things you can legally put into your body. Artificial fats are created by chemically inserting hydrogen—hence the name "hydrogenated" or "partially hydrogenated" fats—into vegetable oils to make them solid at room temperature.[q] Trans fats/partially hydrogenated oil are primarily found in vegetable shortening, margarine, ready-made baked goods and pastries, and fried foods and snacks.

Trans fats are stable and hard to break down, which is why they increase the shelf life of food but decrease yours. Trans fats cause systemic inflammation in your body, incorporate themselves into your blood vessels, and harden your arteries. No other food does more to raise your risk of heart disease. For

---

q   Ruminants like cows, goats, and sheep produce a type of natural trans fat called vaccenic acid which is contained in their fat and dairy. Vaccenic acid has a different chemical structure than industrial trans fats and seems to have the opposite effect on health: in the same studies that found that industrial trans fats shorten your lifespan, the ruminant trans fat *lowered* the risk of diabetes.[261]

every 2 percent increase in calories from trans fats in your diet, your chances of getting heart disease shoot up by 23 percent.[296] In two studies over a period of seven to ten years, the risk of dying from *any* cause (the so-called all-cause mortality) was 34 percent higher for people who consumed the most trans fats compared to people who consumed the least.[261] According to the World Health Organization, trans fats are "a toxic chemical that kills," causing 500,000 premature deaths per year.[297]

As you can imagine, eating trans fats during pregnancy isn't good for your baby either. Irish researchers tracked mothers' diets during pregnancy. The children of mothers who ate the most margarine and spreadable fat had a 66–88 percent higher rate of asthma by age three.[228] A set of German studies found similar results when mothers consumed a lot of margarine or vegetable oils in the last four weeks of pregnancy.[226] Likewise, children who mainly ate margarine rather than butter in the first two years of life had a 90 percent increase in eczema risk and double the rate of allergies.[227]

The World Health Organization has called for a global ban of trans fats from food products, and regulators are finally starting to follow suit. The US Food and Drug Administration has banned them as of June 2018, though some products manufactured before this date can still be sold until 2021.[298] This ban is estimated to save the United States $140 billion in healthcare costs over the next twenty years.[299] In Europe, some countries like Denmark, Sweden, and Switzerland have banned trans fats, while most others have merely introduced weak labelling laws. Wherever you are, if you see trans fats, "partially hydrogenated" oils, or "hardened" vegetable oils on an ingredient label, steer clear.

CHAPTER 6

HOW SUGAR CAUSES OBESITY AND CHRONIC DISEASE

Almost all adults in Western countries consume more sugar than is healthy, and children and teenagers even consume two to three times more than the recommended limit. The World Health Organization recommends that less than 10 percent, and ideally no more than 5 percent, of our daily caloric intake should come from added sugars.[300] For adults, that works out to a maximum of about six teaspoons of added sugar per day, and for children—depending on their age and weight—a lot less. And yet, when American toddlers reach the tender age of nineteen months, their sugar intake has been jacked up to a dose that would be too high even for adults: on average, they consume more than seven teaspoons of added sugar per day.[301] British toddlers aren't far behind.[302]

The culprit is our Western junk food diet. Processed foods are laden with cheap, inflammatory vegetable oils and added sugar. The key word here is "added": it means sugars that don't occur naturally in the food but have been added to the food or drink by the manufacturer. A tablespoon of ketchup contains one tea-spoon of added sugar; a can of sugar-sweetened soda contains ten![300] It quickly adds up, and it's everywhere. About 80 percent of packaged foods in the United States now contain cheap, added sugars, often in the form of high-fructose corn syrup.[303] A common trick that food manufacturers like to use is to add many different types of sugars in small amounts, so that individually, they are listed at the end of the ingredient list. If you added them all up, "sugar" would be listed first among the main ingredients. Food manufacturers also like to use wholesome-sounding names like agave nectar, concentrated apple or grape juice, cane juice crystals, treacle, or various syrups (corn, malt, rice, carob, and golden). Other names for sugar end in "-ose": fructose, glucose, maltose, sucrose, and lactose.

As a result of these efforts, global per-capita intake of sugar has increased by 50 percent in the last fifty years. The one-two punch of cheap vegetable oils and added sugars is the driving force behind the global obesity and diabetes epidemic. Since 1980, worldwide obesity rates have doubled, and diabetes rates have quadrupled.[304,305] And of course, avoiding these chronic conditions isn't just worth it for the mother but also for the child: being obese or diabetic during pregnancy raises the risk that the child will develop asthma, eczema, and allergies.

To explain how sugar leads to inflammation in your body, let's take one step back and look at what your body does with car-bohydrates (or carbs for short). Carbohydrates are sugary or starchy foods such as bread, pasta, rice, cake, potatoes, grains, and of course sugar in any form. Carbohydrate foods are made up of chains of sugars. Based on the length of these sugar chains, carbs are divided into "simple" and "complex" carbs. Simple carbohydrates have only one or two sugar units in the chain, so they break down easily during digestion and quickly enter your bloodstream. This makes your blood sugar levels shoot up. Examples of foods with simple carbohydrates include:

- Sugars; sugary foods and drinks like candy, soda, and most packaged cereals; and fruit juices.
- Highly refined flours and starches like white bread, white pasta, white rice, cakes, and pastries.[r]

Complex carbs, on the other hand, have three or more sugar units in the chain, so they take longer to break down during digestion. Therefore, they are slower to enter your bloodstream and slower to raise your blood sugar levels. When we talk about complex carbs, we mean foods like whole-grain bread, pasta, rice, and cereals, whole fruits and vegetables, and legumes like beans and peas. These complex carbs are rich in fibre, which—as you saw in chapter 4—feed your beneficial bacteria and keep your gut healthy.

When you eat carbs, your body breaks the sugar chains down into glucose, also known as blood sugar. Glucose is the body's primary fuel. As the glucose enters your bloodstream, your pancreas releases insulin. This hormone serves two purposes: carrying the glucose into your cells, where it can be used as fuel, and regulating the amount of glucose in your blood. Too much glucose can be toxic; too little and your cells can't get the fuel they need. When you have more glucose in your blood than your cells can take in, the excess gets carried off by insulin to be stored in the liver and muscles as glycogen—and when energy is needed, glycogen gets converted back to glucose and

---

r   Technically, flours and starches are complex carbs because they contain three or more linked sugar units. But because your body breaks them down as quickly as simple carbs, with the same rapid effect on blood sugar, they are in practice classed as simple carbs.

released into your bloodstream. However, when the liver's glycogen stores are full, excess glucose is converted to fatty acids and stored as fat, particularly in the belly, buttocks, thighs, and breasts. And when *those* fat stores are full, the fatty acids begin to spill over into your organs, like heart, liver, and kidney.

Hence, when you eat lots of sugar or simple carbs, your blood sugar levels spike rapidly, and your pancreas floods your bloodstream with insulin to bring them back down to normal levels. As a result, after a short burst of energy, your blood sugar levels crash, and you feel tired, hungry, and craving a sugary pick-me-up, coffee, or energy drink. When you give in to this craving, the blood sugar roller coaster starts again: spike, crash, repeat. Along the way, the excess glucose accumulates as fat, and you slowly gain weight.

FROM SUGAR TO INFLAMMATION AND GESTATIONAL DIABETES

So how does sugar affect your immune system and inflammation? First, immediately after eating sugary foods, the spike in blood sugar levels dampens your immune system's ability to fight infections. When your blood sugar level is high, your white blood cells—whose job it is to engulf and gobble up harmful bacteria as well as dead or damaged cells in a process called phagocytosis—get sluggish. In one study, volunteers consumed 100 g/3.5 oz of sugar (the equivalent of about two and a half cans of Coca-Cola). Within one to two hours, their ability to fight infections through phagocytosis was reduced by about 50 percent and only recovered slowly over the next five to six hours.[306] Thus, consuming sugar directly increases your odds of getting sick, and perhaps needing antibiotics, by lowering your immune system activity.

Your body's second immediate reaction to sugar consumption, especially to fructose, is to release inflammatory cytokines— in other words, unleash inflammation.[307,308] Fructose is also particularly taxing for your liver. That's why some researchers believe that, out of the various sugars in our diet, fructose is the main culprit behind the rise in obesity, diabetes, and heart disease.[309,310] It's also why high-fructose corn syrup is worse for you than other sugars, and so is—despite its marketing as a health food—agave nectar, which is 85 percent fructose (plain sugar is only 50 percent fructose).[311] And it's why drinking lots of fruit juice, which is loaded with fructose but lacking any of the beneficial fibre of the whole fruit, is a bad idea. Did you know that fruit juices contain about the same amount of sugar as Coca-Cola?[312] Sure, they contain a few more vitamins than soft drinks, but they're really not healthy for you. Smoothies, especially when homemade, retain the beneficial fibre, so they're better—and whole fruit is best.

Third, as always with diet, it comes back to your gut bacteria. High-sugar diets promote the growth of bad bacteria and yeasts like *C. difficile*, *C. perfringens*, and *Candida*,[313,314] which in children are linked to a higher risk of developing asthma, eczema, and allergies.[54,315,316] Indeed, a study of nearly 9,000 mothers in the UK found that when the mothers ate a high amount of sugar during pregnancy, their children had a roughly 75 percent increased risk of asthma and a 30 percent increased risk of allergies by age seven to nine.[317]

These are just the direct effects of sugar on your health. There are indirect ones, resulting from the body fat packed on by eating too much sugar and carbs. As you've seen, your body converts excess blood sugar to fat. This body fat doesn't just sit there like a squishy, silent blanket; instead, it acts like an "endocrine organ" which releases a constant stream of inflammatory cytokines and hormones.[318] This is why being overweight or obese leads to long-term inflammation and all of the chronic health problems that come with it.

On a side note, here's an interesting bit of trivia: the number of fat cells in your body gets set during childhood, and after that, their number can only go up, never down.[319,320] When you gain weight, the fat cells fill up, and you may also develop new ones. When you lose weight, the fat cells get squeezed dry, but they don't disappear—they are still there. What's more, they're sending signals to your body begging for food so they can fill up again, which is why it's so hard to lose weight permanently and avoid the yo-yo effect. Before I got pregnant, I never struggled with my weight. Then, during pregnancy, I gained about twenty pounds, and it has been really tough to get rid of it; five years later, I'm still about five pounds heavier than I used to be. But if body fat acts like a supervillain, muscle mass is the superhero that fights it. Like fat, muscle mass is an endocrine organ, and it counteracts fat by releasing anti-inflammatory and fat-burning substances.[321]

The most immediate danger for your pregnancy posed by a high-sugar/carb diet and by being overweight is developing gestational diabetes. Being overweight doubles your risk of gestational diabetes, and being obese nearly quadruples it.[322] Along with the rise of obesity, the prevalence of gestational diabetes has nearly doubled in the last twenty years and now affects roughly one in ten pregnancies in the United States.[323] Gestational diabetes happens when your blood sugar levels during pregnancy are too high. Normally, your pancreas produces insulin to manage blood sugar levels. During pregnancy, however, the placenta releases hormones which have an insulin-blocking effect. Thus, your body has to manufacture more insulin to keep your blood sugars at a healthy level. When you are eating high-sugar/carb foods, the pancreas may not be able to keep up sufficient insulin production, leading to gestational diabetes.

Gestational diabetes can have serious consequences when it is not treated properly with diet and exercise. It raises the mother's risk of preeclampsia, a high blood pressure condition that is a leading cause of death for both pregnant women and babies worldwide.[324] About half of the women diagnosed with gestational diabetes will go on to develop type 2 diabetes in the five to ten years after birth, which is a seven times higher risk than for women who have not had gestational diabetes.[325] For the baby, gestational diabetes nearly doubles the risk for eczema and food allergies.[326]

SOME SUGARS ARE BETTER, AND ARTIFICIAL SWEETENERS ARE WORSE

Are some sugars better than others? Yes, definitely. In our kitchen, we only use honey, maple syrup, and occasionally molasses as sweeteners. The rawer and more unrefined, the better. As a rule of thumb, the darker the honey or maple syrup, the more antioxidants and nutrients it contains.

Honey has been used as a medicine since ancient times, possibly as long as 8,000 years ago, due to its strong antibacterial, antifungal, and antiviral properties. Good-quality, unrefined honey contains up to 200 different antioxidant compounds like flavonoids, phenolic acids, tocopherols, and ascorbic acid. Ancient cultures in Egypt, Assyria, China, Greece, and Rome used it for wound healing and treating intestinal diseases.[327] In the last few decades, dozens of studies have examined the medical properties of honey. Several of them found that unlike regular sugar, which triggers inflammation, honey actually decreases inflammation. In two studies, consuming some high-quality (natural, unprocessed) honey daily for a few weeks lowered blood markers of inflammation by about 3–7 percent.[328,329] Not too shabby for something so tasty! It also lowers "bad" (LDL) cholesterol and raises "good" (HDL) cholesterol, which makes it useful in dealing with diabetes and heart disease.[328–332] There are even signs that honey is effective in cancer prevention and treatment.[333,334] An important reminder, though—honey should never be given to children under one year of age. Honey can be contaminated with *Clostridium botulinum* spores (dormant bacteria), which in rare cases can trigger a dangerous poisoning that affects a baby's nervous system, so-called infant botulism. For what it's worth, I don't think children under one should be given *anything* that's sweetened with *any* kind of sugar, other than naturally sweet fruit!

Compared to honey, there is less research on the benefits of maple syrup, and so far, the research has only been in vitro (experiments on individual cells in a test tube) rather than in vivo (tests in living humans or animals). Nonetheless, these lab experiments show that maple syrup contains a good amount of antioxidants and bioactive compounds[335,336] and that these can slow the growth of colon and breast cancer cells.[337–339] If you buy maple syrup, choose the darkest grade you can find.

With all that said, remember that honey and maple syrup are still sugars which raise your blood sugar levels, and that's something you'd rather avoid. I wouldn't recommend eating *more* sweet foods just because they contain honey or maple syrup; I would only use them as healthier options to *replace* cane sugar and other sweeteners.

You may wonder about artificial sweeteners like aspartame (brand names: NutraSweet, Equal, Canderel), saccharin (Sweet'N Low, Sugar Twin, Sweet Twin, Sweetex, Natreen), sucralose (Splenda), acesulfame-K (Sunett, Sweet One), or cyclamate (banned in the United States but allowed in Europe and Canada; Sweet'N Low, Sugar Twin, Natreen). Since they don't contain any carbs or calories, are they a good option? Unfortunately, the answer is a hard no.

Artificial sweeteners have been marketed as healthy sugar substitutes and weight-loss helpers for decades, but frequent consumers of them are more likely to become obese and diabetic.[340] How is that possible? There are four reasons why this happens:

1. Food activates a reward system in the human brain. This reward system has two parts: the first one gets triggered by the taste of food, the second by the compounds released when the food gets broken down by digestion. Artificial sweeteners fire up the first part of the reward system (taste) but not the second (digestion), because there *is* nothing to digest, so the reward system stays active and unfulfilled. This drives us to search for more food to satisfy the second part of the reward system. Therefore, rather than reducing our overall calorie consumption, artificial sweeteners make us feel more hungry and search for more calories, and thus make us gain weight.[340]

2. The more we eat certain flavours, the more we learn to like them. Supposedly "guilt-free" artificial sweeteners train our preference for sweeter and sweeter foods and drinks, and thus increase our sugar cravings—again leading to more obesity and diabetes.[340]

3. Because artificial sweeteners decouple sweet taste from cal-

ories, they mess with our body's delicate balance between blood sugar levels and insulin.[341] When we taste something sweet, our body expects carbs and a rise in blood sugar, so it releases insulin.[342] The blood sugar spike never comes, and over time, the body adapts and dials down its insulin response to sweet-tasting foods and drinks. Then, when we consume *actual* carbs and sugar, the body releases less insulin, and our blood sugar spikes even higher than usual, which results in inflammation and fat accumulation.

4. A bombshell study published in *Nature* in 2014 demonstrated that artificial sweeteners harm the gut microbiome even more so than sugar. They reduce the number of anti-inflammatory *Lactobacillus* bacteria while promoting bacteria associated with diabetes in humans. The study demonstrated that these changes directly cause glucose intolerance—a state of permanently elevated blood sugar levels which lead to diabetes.[343,344]

As you can see, most of these issues—messing with our reward and insulin systems and acquiring a preference for sweeter flavours—also apply to "natural" zero-calorie sweeteners like stevia. Personally, I think stevia tastes pretty awful, so I'm more than happy to avoid it. Another popular "natural" sweetener is xylitol, a sugar alcohol. It's not zero-calorie—it has 33 percent fewer calories than regular sugar but tastes very similar and barely raises blood sugar levels. However, because xylitol can't be broken down completely in our digestive system, it gives many people severe bloating, flatulence, and diarrhoea. Supposedly this is temporary and goes away if you consume xylitol regularly, but let's just say we tried and can't confirm. Xylitol is definitely not something you should use on a first date.

We are slowly discovering that the food additives in processed food—not just artificial sweeteners—wreak havoc on our microbiome.[345] We still know very little about how the hundreds of permitted food additives interact with our microbiome, but what we already *do* know is looking pretty bad.[346-348] For example, in the late 1990s, food companies started adding trehalose—a type of sugar naturally occurring in mushrooms, yeasts, and shellfish—to act as a stabiliser in ready meals, TV dinners, and processed foods. Trehalose keeps foods moist and improves their texture. You'll find it in everything from cookies to chewing gum to nutrition bars to ground beef. Now it turns out that trehalose specifically fosters the growth of the most virulent strains of antibiotic-resistant *Clostridium difficile*—and very likely helped kick-start the growing *C. difficile* epidemic which kills about 30,000 people in the United States every year.[349] Likewise, the ubiquitous food thickener maltodextrin has been found to promote the growth of *E. coli* and simultaneously thin the mucus barrier in our gut, probably contributing to the rise of Crohn's and other inflammatory bowel diseases.[350]

In sum, processed foods contain inflammatory fats, sugars, and chemical additives, all of which foster the growth of harmful microbes. So the recent findings that our body reacts to processed foods just as it would react to a bacterial infection really aren't that surprising![281,351,352]

HOW TO KEEP YOUR BLOOD SUGARS UNDER CONTROL

Keeping your blood sugars in check is pretty straightforward, once you know how. Avoid processed foods, especially refined grains like white bread, white rice, pasta, pastries, and sugary foods and drinks. Instead, eat whole foods that are naturally high in dietary fibre, like vegetables, legumes, fruits, and whole grains. The fibre slows down carbohydrate digestion and thus avoids blood sugar spikes—and it will feed your beneficial gut microbes.

Next, add good fats to your meals. Be liberal with the olive oil, throw avocados into your smoothies, have nut butters on your whole-grain bread. Not only does fat make the food taste more satisfying, but it will also slow down carbohydrate digestion and blood sugar release. That's because the fat slows down gastric emptying—the rate at which food passes from the stomach to the intestines, where the nutrients are absorbed into the bloodstream.

Try to literally "eat the rainbow" by choosing colourful foods: berries, pomegranate, brightly coloured vegetables, herbs, spices like cinnamon and turmeric, olives and olive oil, and—not during pregnancy, otherwise in moderation—dark chocolate, coffee, and red wine. Antioxidant-rich foods like these lower your blood sugar levels by inhibiting carbohydrate digestion and glucose absorption.[353-355] Besides, as you recall, they are anti-inflammatory and feed the beneficial bacteria in your microbiome.

Most importantly, though, you don't need to feel deprived. Eating healthy foods that keep your blood sugars in check doesn't have to be joyless. As with my recommendation for how to incorporate good fats and fibre in your meals, I'd turn to the Mediterranean diet—it's simple, joyful, and tasty.

You don't even have to miss out on sweet treats. Here are some of our favourites:

- Dried Medjool dates with almond butter—a perfect combination of creamy, chewy, sweet, nutty, and a bit of crunch!

- Freeze some chopped banana, then blend it with almond butter, cinnamon, and a touch of maple syrup and sea salt for a super-tasty homemade ice cream.
- A super-simple snack: have some slices of apple with almond butter or dark tahini (ground roasted sesame seeds).
- Make buckwheat pancakes (the French call them *galettes*) with tahini and a drizzle of honey. The pancake batter is just buckwheat flour, water, and salt in a thin mixture that covers a spoon but drizzles off it easily. These pancakes are also great smothered with homemade jam—simply blend some frozen berries, some dates for sweetness, and chia seeds for a jammy texture.

None of these treats takes more than five to ten minutes to make, and they are so good you won't believe it. Our daughter gobbles them up, and we don't mind because they're all healthy.

YOUR BABY'S DEVELOPING TASTE BUDS

This seems like a good time to bring up the relationship between your diet, especially during pregnancy and breastfeeding, and your baby's developing taste buds. In short, what you eat during these times will influence what flavours your child will like as it grows up.

Both the amniotic fluid in your womb and your breast milk take on the flavours of what you ate a few hours before. From fifteen to sixteen weeks of age, the foetus begins to respond to the flavour of the amniotic fluid—guzzling more when it tastes sweet, and less when it tastes bitter.[356] Babies that are exposed to vegetables, herbs, spices, and other strong flavours in the womb or through breast milk like those flavours more in childhood and later in life. In contrast, babies who are formula-fed learn to prefer its relatively bland and sweet flavour and are less accepting of new flavours and foods during weaning.[357,358] Studies with rats also indicate that if you indulge in junk food during pregnancy and breastfeeding, your baby will learn to like these flavours, too, and is more likely to end up obese later in life.[359]

By putting a bit more work into your diet during pregnancy and breastfeeding, you are less likely to have a picky eater on your hands later. This means less stress and fewer battles at mealtimes. It also gives your child the gift of taste preferences that can keep them healthy throughout their entire life and establish a love of discovering new flavours and cuisines.

Our daughter has always loved strong and even sour flavours—I suspect because I was addicted to cranberry juice during pregnancy. Some of her favourites are steamed broccoli or artichokes dipped in balsamic vinegar, crunchy sauerkraut, garlic beans with lots of peppery olive oil, earthy cooked beetroot, acidic green olives, spicy ginger and lemon tea, or green smoothies with avocado, kale, and parsley. She hoovers up bowls of berries that I personally find too sour. As a toddler, she loved sardines straight from the tin, which I can only stomach with mayo. We've recently started introducing Korean food, and now she keeps asking for kimchi rice. Of course, like every kid, she has days where she's refusing foods or demanding plain rice, bread, or pasta, but she is generally happy to try new flavours—especially if she spots something on Mama's or Papa's plate that's not on hers.

CHAPTER 7

SUPPLEMENTS BEFORE, DURING, AND AFTER PREGNANCY

Let's talk about supplements. You may wonder whether you should be taking any to support your growing baby. In short, yes, but you shouldn't see it as a replacement for a healthy, balanced diet. While healthy food is more work, it provides a much bigger variety and higher quality of nutrients and antioxidants than any pill, and it creates better lifelong habits and flavour preferences for your child. Time and time again, studies have confirmed that a varied, healthy whole-foods diet during pregnancy—which delivers a broad range of vitamins and antioxidants—makes it less likely that your child will suffer from chronic diseases.[360] If I had to pick a single diet based on tastiness, health benefits, and ease of preparation, it would be the Mediterranean diet. I have talked about its benefits multiple times in this book: among them is a dramatic reduction in asthma, allergy, and other atopic diseases.[184,361]

Yet, medical research has also zeroed in on a number of *specific* nutrients that play a role in preventing both atopic diseases and neurodevelopmental disorders. This is where supplements can play an extremely useful role.

As soon as I was trying to get pregnant, I began taking a range of supplements to complement my diet. My goal was to start building up the nutrient stores in my body before pregnancy. Minerals generally get stored in the skeleton, teeth, muscles, and some organs, while iron builds up in the blood. Some vitamins—the fat-soluble ones—get stored in the liver and fat tissue, while any water-soluble vitamins not used up by the body are peed out quickly.[362] These nutrient stores are depleted during pregnancy, so if you are planning to have a second child, you would ideally wait at least twenty-four months before getting pregnant again to allow your body to rebuild its nutrient stores. This lowers the risk of preterm births, low birthweight, and infant mortality for the second baby.[363]

So which supplements are worth taking? Each woman's needs are slightly different, and you may want to talk with your healthcare provider about whether you are deficient in any particular nutrient. The list below is not exhaustive—these aren't the *only* nutrients you need, but they are essential ones that are both commonly deficient and involved in the prevention of chronic illnesses. You can find a summary of all the nutrients and their benefits discussed in this chapter in appendix 2, as well as up-to-date links to supplements at **www.growhealthybabies.com/supplements**.

FOLATE (VITAMIN B9)

Folate is one of the most critical nutrients in early pregnancy. It's required for the development of your baby's neural tube in the first twenty-eight days after conception. The neural tube is the part of the embryo that will later turn into the brain and spinal cord. A sufficient supply of folate is necessary to prevent birth defects like spina bifida (incomplete closing of the backbone and membrane around the spinal cord), anencephaly (incomplete development of major parts of the brain), cleft lip and palate, as well as premature birth, low birth weight, and miscarriage.[364,365] Besides preventing birth defects, the benefits of taking folate in the first trimester last well into childhood: by four years of age, children exposed to folate early in pregnancy have higher verbal function and social competence, and by age eight, they suffer less from hyperactivity and problems with peers.[366,367]

However, about 10 percent of women suffer from a condition in which their bodies accumulate excessive amounts of folate, potentially leading to serious health problems. Why is that, and how would you know if you were one of these women? It turns out that *I am* one of them, and I found out purely by chance.

When Victor and I were still living in London, we had been trying to conceive for over a year, and I had also suffered two very early miscarriages. My GP took a blood test and noticed a small abnormality in my hormone profile, so she referred me to a fertility clinic at University College London. The doctors there discovered that I had a not-that-uncommon genetic mutation on a gene called MTHFR—up to 12 percent of the population in Western countries have it.[368] When you have this mutation, your body cannot properly metabolise folate. Thus, it can accumulate in your body and cause all sorts of problems.[369]

In case you're curious, the box titled "The MTHFR Mutation" provides some more details on the MTHFR mutation and its implications.

THE MTHFR MUTATION

MTHFR stands for "methylene tetrahydrofolate reductase," which is quite a mouthful. The mutation is linked to some serious health problems–an increased risk of heart disease, colon cancer, stroke, recurrent miscarriage, Alzheimer's disease, and depression–so I just started calling it the "motherf***** gene."

The MTHFR gene instructs the body to create the MTHFR enzyme. When you have the MTHFR mutation, your body produces between 20-70 percent less of the MTHFR enzyme. This enzyme is needed to convert folate (whether from food or supplements) into L-methylfolate, the biologically active form that our body can use. Thus, the MTHFR mutation means that you will be deficient in L-methylfolate.

L-methylfolate, in turn, is crucial for the process of DNA methylation (that's the process we discussed in the epigenetics section of chapter 2). DNA methylation is how unnecessary, unwanted, or potentially harmful genes are silenced during gene expression, which keeps our "cellular factories" running smoothly and prevents chronic diseases.

At the same time, when your body can't convert the folate you're consuming–and especially when you're taking folic acid supplements during pregnancy–the unmetabolised folate can accumulate in your body and lead to liver damage, reduced immune function, and a heightened risk of some cancers.

Fortunately, there *is* a solution. You can buy supplements that contain L-methylfolate, the biologically active form of folate that your body can use directly. Unfortunately, they are more expensive than regular folic acid supplements. You also need to stick to the dose recommended on the packaging. L-methylfolate bypasses the body's built-in safeguards against over-methylation, which can cause side effects like sore muscles, irritability, anxiety, and others.[370] The brands that I use are BioCare Liquid Methylfolate and Metagenics FolaPro, but there are several to choose from (sometimes the L-methylfolate is labelled or branded differently, e.g., as L-5-methylfolate, 5-MTHF, Metafolin, or Quatrefolic)–see also **www.growhealthybabies.com/supplements.**

The only way to find out for sure if you have the MTHFR mutation is to take a genetic test. If your doctor can't or won't order a test for you, you could use genetic home-testing kits like 23andMe or Color. But genetic tests aren't cheap, and maybe you're also concerned about the privacy implications. Either way, whether you *know* that you have the MTHFR mutation, or whether you *don't know* but want to be sure that your body can metabolise the folate supplements, you can take the L-methylfolate supplements mentioned above. They are fine to use whether you have the MTHFR mutation or not, as long as you stick to the recommended dose–but discuss it with your doctor to be sure.

On a side note, a lack of folate is also involved in fertility problems. One of the most common reasons for infertility–about 20 percent of cases–is failure to ovulate.[371] Taking folate supplements reduces the risk of ovulatory failure drastically, so my doctor in London suspected that my body's inability to process folic acid, due to the MTHFR mutation, could be causing my fertility problems. They recommended that I try the L-methylfolate supplement, and bam–two months later, I was pregnant.

In summary, whether you have the MTHFR mutation or not, it's definitely a good idea to take folic acid or L-methylfolate (see "The MTHFR Mutation" for more info) supplements as soon as you are trying to get pregnant. How much should you be taking? The US Preventive Services Task Force recommends a **daily supplement of 400–800 µg.**[372]

You can also get natural folate from foods. Good dietary sources are:

- Lentils, beans, and chickpeas (230–350 µg per cup)
- Asparagus, kale, and spinach (260–270 µg per cup)
- Turnip greens/leaves and broccoli (170 µg per cup)
- Avocado (120 µg per cup)

VITAMIN D

Vitamin D is essential to keeping your bones and teeth healthy and also plays a crucial role in regulating the immune system. Your main source of vitamin D is sunshine—literally. Your skin makes vitamin D through a chemical reaction that is triggered by exposure to sunlight, specifically light in the ultraviolet B (UVB) spectrum.

Vitamin D deficiency is also, in the words of Harvard Medical School researchers, "the single most important dietary deficiency in the world today"—linked to prostate cancer, colon cancer, breast cancer, and now increasingly asthma and allergies.[373] If you are lacking vitamin D, you are more prone to getting colds and other infections. Your body is also more likely to mistakenly turn the immune system's weapons on itself and develop autoimmune conditions like multiple sclerosis, rheumatoid arthritis, diabetes, inflammatory bowel disease, and lupus.[374] It's no surprise, then, that vitamin D is hugely important during pregnancy as well. Researchers have found positive effects of supplementing vitamin D on many different chronic diseases and health outcomes.

For starters, a lack of vitamin D increases the risk of gestational diabetes by nearly 50 percent (which in turn nearly doubles your child's risk of eczema and food allergies, as we saw in the previous chapter on sugar). Being deficient in vitamin D also increases the likelihood of preeclampsia—a leading cause of death for both pregnant women and babies—by 70 percent.[375]

Due to its importance for the immune system, allergy researchers suspect that taking vitamin D during pregnancy can help prevent asthma, eczema, and allergies; however, the findings so far have been mixed. What is clear from numerous studies is that children who have these chronic diseases are generally deficient in vitamin D. In the case of asthma, taking vitamin D supplements decreases the severity of asthma symptoms in children who already have the disease: it roughly cuts the number of asthma attacks and hospital visits in half.[376-379] Likewise, several—but not all—studies show that when mothers take vitamin D during pregnancy, it reduces the occurrence of wheezing and asthma symptoms in their children.[361,380,381] The same goes for eczema: vitamin D appears to lower eczema symptoms in children who have the disease.[377] One Japanese study found that taking vitamin D during pregnancy significantly decreased children's eczema risk,[380] but others didn't find such a link.[381,382]

How much vitamin D should you take? In the United States, the official recommended daily allowance (RDA) is set at 600 IU[s] per day for adults, including pregnant or breastfeeding

---

s   "IU" stands for "International Units"—a measure of potency, or biological activity, rather than a weight.

women. This dose is designed to achieve sufficient vitamin D blood levels of 50 nanomoles per litre (nmol/L).

However, it turns out that the official RDA might be much too low. A team of Canadian researchers recently discovered that this recommendation is based on a statistical error. According to their calculations, a dose more than ten times higher—8,900 IU per day—would be needed to achieve those vitamin D blood levels.[383] Other experts confirmed their calculations and are now calling on public health authorities to **raise the RDA to 7,000 IU** per day. Up to 10,000 IU per day is considered safe.[384,385]

Personally, I took 6,000 IU per day in liquid form from a spray. Just don't overdo it—vitamin D can become toxic at long-term doses of over 10,000 IU per day. For comparison, if you're fair-skinned (or ghostly white, like me), your body will produce about 20,000 IU from half an hour of full-body sun exposure.[386]

IRON

Every single cell in the human body needs iron, and it needs the right amount—both too little and too much iron can be harmful.[387] Among other things, iron is required in making and repairing DNA and in producing haemoglobin, the red blood cells which transport oxygen around your body. Yet, iron deficiency is surprisingly common—it is one of the most widespread nutrient deficiencies in the world and affects 30–50 percent of all pregnancies.

Iron also plays a role in balancing the immune system. It shifts the activity of T-helper cells from Th2 back to Th1—and as we saw in chapter 1, an immune system stuck in Th2 mode is the trigger for allergies and atopic disease. A British study involving 2,000 mothers, which tracked their children's health for ten years after birth, found that iron deficiency in the first trimester—when the lungs begin to develop—makes it about 35 percent more likely that the child will develop lung problems and wheezing. Likewise, when mothers are iron-deficient at the time of giving birth, their child's probability of developing allergies goes up by about 30 percent.[388]

Iron is even more crucial to normal brain development. Iron deficiency during pregnancy and the first few years of life leads to changes in the brain's structure, its neurotransmitters (the chemicals that transmit signals throughout the brain and body), and its myelination (the insulation around its wiring and connections). Most researchers believe that these changes are permanent and irreversible.[387,389]

The effects of iron deficiency during pregnancy and early childhood are well-documented. They include lower scores on nearly every measure of mental development—cognitive function and learning ability, language, recognizing their mother's voice or face, social-emotional function, lower moods and attention-deficit hyperactivity disorder (ADHD), or motor control. A study of Costa Rican teens that had been severely iron deficient as infants—and were subsequently treated with iron supplements—found that they still scored lower on cognitive tests at age nineteen compared to teens who hadn't been iron deficient. The reverse is also true: children who had higher blood levels of haemoglobin (which depends on iron supply) at six months of age achieved higher IQ scores later in life. At age five, each increase of 10 g haemoglobin per litre of blood resulted in 1.75 points higher IQ scores.[390,391]

The US National Institutes of Health's **RDA is 27 mg/day during pregnancy** and **9 mg/day during breastfeeding**.[392] Given the importance of iron for brain development, I personally aimed to consume more than the RDA. It's generally safe, but mild side effects like an upset tummy or constipation can occur at levels above 45 mg/day. Iron only becomes toxic at much higher doses—about 5 mg per pound of body weight, or about 750 mg/ day for a 150-pound woman.

Other than supplements, where can you get iron in your diet? There are two forms: heme iron (from animals) and non-heme iron (from plants). Heme iron is more easily absorbed by your body, but non-heme iron is easier to digest because the plant sources also contain fibre—which feeds your microbiome, so it's a double win. Vitamin C increases the absorption of non-heme iron by a factor of three, while calcium prevents iron absorption—so if you want to maximise your iron uptake, avoid calcium supplements (and dairy) alongside iron-rich foods or iron supplements.[393,394]

Below is a list of good dietary sources and their iron content per serving.[392,395]

Non-heme (plant-based) iron:

- Soybeans (8 mg per cup) and tofu (5 mg per cup)
- Lentils (7 mg per cup)
- Spinach (6 mg per cup)
- Sesame seeds and tahini (5 mg per ¼ cup, or a whopping 20 mg per cup)
- All types of beans and chickpeas (4 mg per cup)
- Olives (4 mg per cup)
- Pumpkin seeds (3 mg per ¼ cup = a small handful, or 12 mg per cup)
- Green leafy vegetables and herbs like swiss chard, beet

greens, collard greens, bok choy, and parsley (2–4 mg per cup)

- Spices like cumin, chilli, and turmeric (1–2 mg per teaspoon)
- Many other vegetables like green peas, asparagus, brussels sprouts, kale, broccoli, cabbage, lettuce, squash, and fennel (1–2 mg per cup)

Heme (animal-based) iron:

- Canned sardines (2mg per can)
- Grass-fed beef or lamb (2 mg per 3.5 oz/100 g serving)
- Roasted chicken or turkey (1 mg per 3.5 oz/100 g serving)
- Eggs (1 mg per egg)

Even if you're not into legumes or greens—try some tahini (sesame cream) with honey, or tahini with olives, on your breakfast bread/cracker. For us, it's such a delicious staple that we sometimes travel with a jar of tahini just so we don't have to live without it!

ZINC

Like iron, the trace mineral zinc is essential to all forms of life on Earth. All living organisms need it for gene expression, cell development, and cell replication. Deficiency is common: the World Health Organization estimates that 31 percent of the world's population is deficient. During pregnancy, a good supply of zinc is necessary for the healthy development of the baby's gut (especially the gut lining and its permeability), immune system, and brain.[396]

A study in Scotland recruited 2,000 healthy pregnant women and tracked, among other things, their zinc intake during pregnancy. Five years later, the researchers followed up with them about their children's health. They discovered a clear relationship between zinc deficiency and asthma: mothers who met or exceeded the RDA reduced their child's asthma risk by about half. There was a link to eczema as well. Meeting the zinc RDA lowered the child's eczema risk slightly and exceeding the RDA reduced it by about a third.[397] A Harvard study of 1,290 mothers and children essentially came to the same conclusion: mothers with the highest zinc consumption had children with just half the asthma risk compared to mothers with the lowest zinc consumption.[398]

The US **RDA for zinc is 11 mg/day during pregnancy** and **12 mg/day during breastfeeding.** If you eat a balanced, varied diet, you will get a good supply of zinc from a number of different sources:

- Grass-fed beef or lamb (4 mg per 3.5 oz/100 g serving)
- Scallops and shrimp (2 mg per 3.5oz/100 g serving)
- Nuts and seeds: sesame seeds/tahini, pumpkin seeds, and cashews (2.5–3 mg per quarter cup)
- Legumes: lentils, chickpeas, and hummus (2.5 mg per cup)
- You'll also find it in mushrooms, leafy green vegetables, squash, peas, asparagus, tofu, yoghurt and milk, and grains like oats and quinoa.

IODINE

Iodine is a mineral that is required to make thyroid hormones. These, in turn, control the body's metabolism—the way your body uses energy. Thyroid hormones influence your body weight, body temperature, breathing, heart rate, muscle strength, menstrual cycles, functioning of the nervous system, immune responses, and more. During pregnancy and infancy, thyroid hormones—and therefore iodine—are critical for the healthy development of your baby's bones, brain, and nervous system.[399,400]

The World Health Organization estimates that 2 billion people worldwide are not consuming enough iodine. In the United States, 7 percent of pregnant women are deficient in iodine, and as much as half of all women are estimated to be below the RDA.[401] The UK is an anomaly among developed countries: it ranks among the top ten most iodine deficient countries in the world—alongside Pakistan, Ethiopia, Sudan, Russia, Afghanistan, Algeria, Angola, Mozambique, and Ghana. On average, British women consume just 64 percent of the recommended daily amount, and consumption has been declining steadily over the last decades.[402]

You most definitely want to avoid being iodine deficient. Even moderate deficiency is known to lower a child's IQ. Serious deficiency leads to severely stunted physical and mental development (a condition previously known as cretinism) and is the world's leading preventable cause of mental retardation. It also increases the risk of spontaneous abortion, reduced birth weight, and infant mortality.[402,403]

The WHO recommends **250 µg of iodine/day during pregnancy** and **290 µg/day during breastfeeding**. Unless you're eating sea vegetables every day, that is a difficult amount to get from your diet alone, so public health authorities recommend that all women take iodine supplements during pregnancy and breastfeeding.[402]

Sea vegetables like kelp, dulse, and wakame are so rich in iodine that you actually have to be careful not to eat *too much* of it. One teaspoon contains 250 µg and covers your RDA. If you ate more than one tablespoon per day, you could easily surpass the tolerable upper limit of 1,000 µg/day, and too much iodine also causes thyroid dysfunction.[399,404] In small amounts, however, dried seaweed flakes are a very tasty and healthy condiment. In Asian countries, they are sprinkled on top of many dishes to add some extra flavour; you can find them in nearly every Asian food store.

Apart from seaweed:

- You can get about half your RDA's worth from a 3.5 oz/100 g serving of cod or (well-cooked!) shellfish.
- A cup of yoghurt or milk provides 70 µg iodine, somewhere between a third and a quarter of your RDA.
- A 3.5 oz/100 g serving of shrimp, sardines, or salmon contains about 32–46 µg, and an egg has 27 µg.
- There are small amounts in vegetables like sweet potatoes, onions, and spinach, or fruit like strawberries, bananas, and cantaloupe.
- And of course, there is iodized salt, which you can find in most supermarkets. On average, one teaspoon of iodized salt should cover your daily need for iodine.[404]

If you are frequently experiencing pregnancy nausea, I have some comforting news for you. In the first twenty weeks, the nausea is actually a sign of a healthy pregnancy and a sufficient supply of iodine in your body, and is linked to a lower risk of spontaneous abortion.[405] Because too much iodine is not healthy for the embryo either, the nausea appears to be the embryo's way of steering you away from iodine-rich foods like meat, dairy, and seafood.[406]

CHOLINE

Choline plays a crucial role in the development of your baby. It influences the growth and division of stem cells and shuts them down when necessary (so-called apoptosis) to prevent uncontrolled growth. It's also required for developing a healthy spinal cord and brain structure, especially in the hippocampus—a brain region associated with long-term memory, learning, emotion regulation, and social interaction.

The US National Academy of Medicine has only issued dietary recommendations for choline since 1998, so it is one of the most recent additions to the list of essential nutrients. It's also a very common deficiency. About 90 percent of the US population is below the recommended daily intake, including 90–95 percent of pregnant women—and most pregnancy supplements don't contain any.[407,408]

Choline deficiency during pregnancy is linked to changes in brain structure that create lifelong memory problems. It can also result in neural tube defects like spina bifida and anencephaly: babies have a four times higher risk of neural tube defects when their mothers have a low-choline diet rather than a high-choline diet. In adults, a chronic lack of choline results in organ dysfunction, muscle damage, mood problems, and memory loss. Choline doesn't just prevent problems: studies show that taking choline supplements can significantly enhance your memory and learning abilities.[408–410]

In the United States, the **recommended daily amount is 450 mg/day during pregnancy** and **550 mg/day during breast-feeding**. Choline is available from many different foods,[411] so if you're eating a healthy, varied diet, you will get a lot of choline without even trying:

- Eggs (150 mg per egg yolk)
- Seafood: shrimp and (well-cooked!) scallops (125–150 mg per 3.5 oz/100 g serving); cod, salmon, and sardines (80–90 mg per 3.5 oz/100 g serving)
- Collard greens, brussels sprouts, and broccoli (60–70 mg per cup)
- Swiss chard, cauliflower, and asparagus (50 mg per cup)
- Peas, spinach, and cabbage (30–40 mg per cup)
- Meat: chicken and turkey (90–100 mg per 3.5 oz/100 g serving); beef (70 mg per 3.5oz/100 g serving)
- Dairy: milk or yoghurt (40 mg per cup)
- You will also get decent amounts from mushrooms, beans, squash, miso/tofu, tomatoes, and other vegetables.

If you're still worried about getting sufficient choline, you can find it in choline-only supplements or commonly also in B-complex vitamins and a few multivitamin products.

As with all supplements, make sure not to overdo it, and consult with your doctor. Side effects of excessive choline begin at about 3,500 mg per day[408] (about seven to eight times the RDA), and range from the merely embarrassing (like fishy body odour and excessive sweating) to the dangerous (low blood pressure and liver toxicity).

VITAMIN E

Vitamin E, also called alpha-tocopherol, is an essential nutrient that supports the health of your eyes, skin, and immune system. Like all antioxidants, it protects your cells and DNA from damage by unstable molecules ("free radicals"). In a balanced diet, a deficiency of vitamin E should be rare—but because of the rise of processed foods, eight out of ten people worldwide and nine out of ten people in America don't consume enough of it.[412-414]

Several studies have pointed to a lack of vitamin E as a risk factor for asthma. In one of these studies, researchers in Scotland tracked the diets of 2,000 healthy pregnant women, then took blood samples to assess their nutrient levels. Five years later, the researchers checked how many of their kids had been diagnosed with asthma. In women with the highest vitamin E consumption, compared to women with the lowest, their children's asthma risk was cut in half.[397] More than half a dozen other studies have come to a similar conclusion.[361]

The **RDA for vitamin E is 15 mg/day during pregnancy** and **19 mg/day during breastfeeding**.[415] It is contained in most pregnancy multivitamins, so you don't usually need a separate supplement.

Vitamin E is also available from a wide variety of foods, especially green leafy vegetables, nuts, seeds, and oil-rich plants like olives and avocados.[416] For example:

- Sunflower seeds (12 mg per ¼ cup = a small handful)
- Almonds (6 mg per ¼ cup) and peanuts (3 mg per ¼ cup)
- Green leafy vegetables: spinach, swiss chard, turnip greens, beet greens, and mustard greens (3–4 mg per cup)
- Vegetables and oily fruit: avocado (3 mg per cup), asparagus (3 mg per cup), broccoli (2 mg per cup), olives (2 mg per cup) and olive oil (2 mg per tablespoon), bell peppers (1–2 mg per cup) and chilli peppers (1–2 mg per teaspoon)
- Fruits and berries: cranberries, raspberries, and kiwi (1 mg per cup)

PROBIOTICS

Your microbiome is key to your health and thus—as you are the initial source of your child's microbiome—the key to your child's health as well. You saw in chapter 2 how gut bacteria modulate and support our immune system and how they influence chronic diseases, inflammation, resistance to infections, even our moods and brain development. In chapters 4–6, we discussed how different foods, fibres, and fats favour the growth of beneficial versus harmful gut bacteria. So what does the research say about probiotic supplements during and after pregnancy, and whether they can help prevent asthma, eczema, and allergies? Quite a lot!

Probiotic supplements can play a major role in eczema prevention. A team of US military doctors reviewed twenty-seven different studies in which probiotics were given to mothers during pregnancy, to infants from birth onwards, or both.[417] On average, they show that probiotics taken by mothers or children in infancy reduce the child's eczema risk by about 25 percent. But that's just the average! Some strains of bacteria are more protective than others: three studies involved *Lactobacillus paracasei*—for the children receiving these bacteria, the eczema risk was cut in half. Probiotics with *Lactobacillus rhamnosus* and mixtures of *Bifidobacteria* also reduce the risk by nearly 50 percent, in some studies even more.

Consider one trial from Japan, where mothers took a mix of *Bifidobacterium longum* and *breve* during the last month of pregnancy, and their babies were given the same mix until the age of six months. A control group of mothers and babies did not receive any probiotics. In this control group, by the age of ten months, 10 out of 31 (32 percent) of the babies had developed eczema—compared to 10 out of *101* (10 percent) of the babies in the probiotic group![418] This means that in this particular study, the probiotics decreased the babies' risk of eczema by nearly 70 percent.

Probiotics can also help to prevent other types of allergic diseases. The risk reduction isn't quite as large as with eczema, but every little bit helps, right? A team of American researchers combed through literally over a thousand studies and combined the results in a meta-analysis, which found that probiotics—either taken during pregnancy or given to your child after birth—reduce your child's risk of developing allergies by 12–14 percent.[419] In some high-risk groups, like kids born via C-section to parents who already have allergies, the risk decreases by as much as 40 percent.[420]

Right now, one particular avenue of research is generating huge excitement in both the medical community and among parents whose kids are affected: the potential of probiotics to not just prevent but *reverse and cure* lethal food allergies. Peanut allergy, for example, is the most common cause of anaphylactic shock—in which the throat and tongue swell rapidly—and the most common cause of death from food allergy.

An Australian trial involved sixty-two children aged one to ten with peanut allergy. Over the course of eighteen months, the children received either a placebo (containing neither peanut nor probiotics) or increasing doses of peanut together with a *Lactobacillus rhamnosus* probiotic. At the end of the trial, 82 percent of kids in the probiotic group were able to eat peanuts without any allergic reaction, compared to just 4 percent of kids in the placebo group![421] When the children were checked again four years later, the majority of those who had received the probiotic were still able to eat peanuts without any problems, and none had experienced an anaphylactic shock.[422]

A similar trial involved babies with cow's milk allergy. For twelve months, they received either hypoallergenic[t] formula with a *Lactobacillus rhamnosus* probiotic or plain hypoallergenic formula without probiotics. When the trial ended, 85 percent of babies in the probiotic group were able to drink cow's milk without any allergic reaction versus just 32 percent in the formula-only group.[423]

Just a note of caution: if you have kids with food allergies and are thinking about a DIY experiment of feeding them the allergen and probiotics—please do *not* try this at home! Anaphylactic shocks are way too dangerous. Oral immunotherapies like these should only be done under medical supervision.

Probiotics are also emerging as an important treatment tool for hay fever, dust allergy, and asthma. More than a dozen studies show that children with these allergic airway diseases experience a strong improvement in their quality of life when they take probiotics. They suffer from fewer allergy and asthma attacks, have a longer time free of symptoms, and their lung function improves.[424-426] There are tantalising signs that probiotics might be able to prevent asthma as well: in high-risk babies that already had eczema and were thus more likely to go on to develop asthma as well, a mix of *Bifidobacterium breve* and prebiotic fibre reduced asthma diagnoses and the need for asthma medication by 20–30 percent.[427] Likewise, in trials with mice, probiotics containing *Lactobacillus rhamnosus* prevented airway inflammation and asthma.[428] However, other studies

---

t   In this "extensively hydrolysed casein formula," the cow's milk protein is broken down into pieces, so babies with cow's milk allergy can safely drink it.

haven't been able to replicate these findings in humans, so there is no definitive evidence *yet* that probiotics alone can prevent asthma.[419,429] Perhaps we simply haven't found the right bacterial strains; more long-term trials are needed.[430]

In addition, probiotics are also proven to lower the risk of gestational diabetes,[431] preeclampsia,[432] premature birth,[433] colds, flus, and other infections,[138,434,435] and mastitis.[136] For me, given their many benefits and well-established safety record (as long as you are not immunocompromised; see chapter 3), taking probiotics has been an obvious choice—I still take them, though not as religiously as I did during my pregnancy and our daughter's first year.

If you choose to take probiotics, here's how to select a good supplement (see also my recommendations at www.growhealthybabies.com/supplements):

- You want as many viable organisms per capsule as possible. Most of the clinical trials mentioned in this book used doses **between 10 billion to 100 billion viable organisms (CFU) per day**. High-quality probiotics have 30–50 billion viable organisms per capsule—I took two capsules containing 30 billion CFU each per day. The cheaper, pharmacy chain-branded probiotics can contain as few as 10 million viable organisms—that's 5,000 times less!
- If you want to give probiotics to your baby or toddler, select a special infant probiotic which contains a different, age-appropriate mix.
- Look for supplements that contain a mix of bacteria, but especially *Lactobacillus rhamnosus* or *paracasei*, and *Bifidobacterium longum, lactis,* or *breve*; these have been found to be most effective in the prevention of atopic diseases.

- Ideally, buy probiotics that have been shipped and stored refrigerated, and store them in the fridge at home.

Remember that *unpasteurised* fermented foods and drinks like yoghurt, sauerkraut, kimchi, kombucha, or kefir are also full of good bacteria (besides many other beneficial nutrients)—about 15 billion organisms per tablespoon. Pasteurised fermented foods are also healthy and tasty, but they lack the living bacteria. You can make fermented foods at home—it's cheap, easy, surprisingly fun, and you can adjust them to your taste. Just search for some recipes online or on YouTube, or check out *The Cultured Club* by Dearbhla Reynolds as well as *The Art of Fermentation* by Sandor Katz. I provide links to these and other recommended books at **www.growhealthybabies.com/books**.

OMEGA-3 FATTY ACIDS AND FISH OIL

We've already covered Omega-3 fatty acids in chapter 5, but they're so important I'll summarise the key facts here again. Fish oils, especially DHA, are the primary building blocks of your child's brain. They are highly anti-inflammatory and help balance your child's developing immune system.

There is plenty of evidence that eating oily fish and supplementing with fish oil capsules during pregnancy reduces your child's risk of atopic diseases. If you do, your child will almost certainly avoid developing food allergies in the first year of life (the risk goes down by nearly 90 percent), be 34 percent less likely to develop any allergies in the first three years of life, and have a 40 percent lower risk of eczema.[234] Children who start eating oily fish before the age of one have a 25 percent reduced risk of asthma and allergies[235] and a good chance of never developing eczema, as the likelihood goes down by 76 percent.[236]

As for brain development, having the Omega-3 fatty acid DHA in your pregnancy diet makes your baby's brain healthier, faster, and more interconnected. This results in better visual perception, eye-hand coordination, motor skills, attention, problem-solving skills, language development, participation in conversation, and significantly higher IQ.[240,241]

Remember that you cannot get a sufficient supply of the relevant Omega-3 fatty acids DHA and EPA from nuts and seeds. They contain an Omega-3 fatty acid called ALA, but your body only converts somewhere between 0–10 percent of it to EPA and DHA.[218,232] If you want to be strictly vegetarian or vegan, you can get EPA and DHA supplements from algae oil.[232]

For pregnant and breastfeeding women, most nutritional guidelines recommend a *minimum* amount of **200–250 mg DHA/ day**.[254] That's about two to three servings of oily fish per week. The best oily fish to add to your diet, based on a combination of high DHA content, sustainability, and low toxicity from environmental pollution, are:

- Anchovies (Atlantic), ca. 900–1,300 mg DHA per 3.5 oz/100 g
- Herring (Atlantic), ca. 1,100–1,200 mg DHA per 3.5 oz/100 g
- Mackerel (Atlantic), ca. 700–900 mg DHA per 3.5 oz/100 g
- Salmon (Pacific), ca. 700–900 mg DHA per 3.5 oz/100 g
- Sardines (Atlantic), ca. 500 mg DHA per 3.5 oz/100 g

In the studies we've discussed in this book, which found beneficial effects of Omega-3 fish oils on brain and immune health, mothers consumed between **400–1,000 mg/day** without any side effects.[255] Personally, I took about 900 mg/day in addition to eating oily fish.

Another important benefit of Omega-3 fish oils is that they can help you beat postpartum depression. However, here is the tricky bit: while DHA is needed for your child's brain development, EPA is the one that can improve your mood.[436] A review of fifteen different trials found that fish oil capsules which contain at least 60 percent EPA, with daily doses between 200–2,200 mg EPA, are an effective treatment against depression. The challenge is that EPA and DHA appear to compete for absorption in your body, and DHA might block the effects of EPA.[437] So if you're taking both, you might want to take them separately at different times, e.g., DHA in the morning and EPA in the evening.

When you decide to take fish oil supplements, it's crucial to choose high-quality brands that are purified, independently tested for heavy metals, and from sustainable sources. The International Fish Oil Standards (IFOS) Program has data for all reputable brands on their website, and LabDoor provides fish oil rankings based on quality and value for money. For more information on fish oil, see **www.growhealthybabies.com/supplements**.

PART III

AVOIDING CHEMICALS: THE CASE FOR ORGANIC AND ECO PRODUCTS

CHAPTER 8

HOW GOING ORGANIC BENEFITS YOUR BABY

If you took away only one thing from reading this book, it should probably be the importance of minding your microbiome. As you saw in chapter 3, that means avoiding unnecessary antibiotic prescriptions. But did you know that the food we eat is constantly exposing us to antibiotics as well? Below, I'll explain how, and what you can do about it.

ANTIBIOTICS IN ANIMAL FARMING

Animal farming is by far the biggest user of antibiotics worldwide. In the United States, more than 80 percent of all antibiotics are given to farm animals. And it's not to protect piglets from sore throats—the antibiotics are used to fatten up the animals so the meat can be produced faster and more cheaply. In a darkly ironic twist, those same antibiotics are coming back to fatten *us* up as well. Researchers now believe that antibiotic residues in farmed meat are contributing to the obesity epidemic in Western societies by tilting our microbiome towards bacteria that disrupt our metabolism and make us obese.[438]

Most antibiotics given to animals are completely unnecessary from a medical point of view, and they add fuel to the fire of the global antibiotic resistance crisis. On US supermarket shelves, more than 80 percent of turkey, 70 percent of pork, 55 percent of ground beef, and 40 percent of chicken contain antibiotic-resistant bacteria like *Salmonella*, *Campylobacter*, and *E. coli*.[439] Farmed fish and shellfish don't fare much better. Around the world, antibiotic use in animal farming is projected to rise by another 67 percent in the next fifteen years, and studies are showing that the more antibiotics are used in farming, the more antibiotic-resistant superbugs spread to humans.[440] Cooking the meat or fish does nothing to inactivate or remove the antibiotic residues,[441] so we're constantly consuming them in small, so-called subtherapeutic, doses. The risks of this have long been well-understood. Consider this warning (issued in 1945, no less!) by Alexander Fleming, the discoverer of penicillin, in his Nobel Prize acceptance lecture: "There is the danger that the ignorant man may easily underdose himself and by exposing his microbes to non-lethal quantities of the drug make them resistant."[442]

How big of a problem is this? The World Health Organization calls antibiotic resistance "one of the biggest threats to global health today."[443] Without efficient antibiotics to combat pathogenic bacteria, medicine could plunge back into a dark age where people routinely died from pneumonia, tuberculosis, or blood infections from even the smallest scratches. This wasn't so long ago—the age of antibiotics only began in 1940.

The first-ever patient to receive an antibiotic—penicillin—was a forty-eight-year-old Oxford police constable named Albert Alexander who had scratched his face working in his rose garden. The scratch became infected with *Streptococci* and *Staphylococci*, and the infection spread to his scalp, shoulder, eyes, and lungs. Albert was on the verge of death when Dr Howard Florey, a pathologist at Oxford University, heard of his case. Florey's lab had been working on turning penicillin into a usable drug—for which Florey would later receive the Nobel Prize together with Fleming. Florey decided to administer the first available doses of penicillin to Alexander, who started to recover. Yet, after five days, Florey's supply ran out. It took 2,000 litres of mould culture to manufacture a single dose of penicillin, and Florey's lab wasn't yet able to manufacture the drug fast enough. Alexander's infection returned with full force, and he died three days later.[444]

This is what our children's future could look like. Alexander's fate is a warning for our own: we were given lifesaving drugs for a while, but they could be taken away from us again. Even worse, we are squandering one of medicine's greatest gifts on cheaper sausages and burgers. Rivers all over the world, including Europe, are "awash with dangerous levels of antibiotics" and farming pesticides, in some cases 300 times over the safe limit.[445,446] A 2016 UK government report estimates that if nothing drastic is done to tackle antibiotic resistance, it will cause 10 million deaths *every year* by 2050.[447]

And this is where organic food comes in—it is farmed without the routine use of antibiotics. It's also much lower in pesticides and has a number of other health benefits.

IS ORGANIC FOOD REALLY HEALTHIER?

In short, yes, it is. Organic food *is* healthier and more nutritious than conventional food.

Two meta-analyses (of 67 and 170 studies, respectively)

demonstrated that organic meat and dairy contain more poly-unsaturated fatty acids than conventional meat and dairy.[448,449] In particular, they contain roughly 50 percent more Omega-3 fatty acids, which—as you saw in chapter 5—are anti-inflammatory and crucial for brain development in children.

The same goes for organic fruit and vegetables. According to a meta-analysis of 343 previous studies, organic produce contains roughly 20–70 percent more antioxidants like phenolic acids, flavanones, stilbenes, flavones, flavonols, and anthocyanins.[450] These prevent DNA and cell damage by neutralising free radicals. Antioxidants have a wide range of health benefits: they lower your risk of cancer, heart disease, age-related eye lens degeneration, and Alzheimer's disease—but only if you get them from your diet, not from supplements. The likely reason is that antioxidants in food are more balanced and complementary than in high-dose supplement antioxidants, as well as having a different chemical composition than industrially produced ones (e.g., there are eight different types of vitamin E in foods but only one type of vitamin E in supplements).[451] It also appears that dietary antioxidants help to balance your gut microbiome.[452] Moreover, organic produce benefits your microbiome in another important way: it provides you with a bigger bacterial diversity because of the higher biodiversity and quality of the soil in which it is grown.[453,454]

But wait a minute. No doubt you have regularly come across articles in the media or on your friends' Facebook feeds, which gleefully "bust the myth" that organic foods are any better for you. Look at those do-gooder hippies overpaying for their precious kale! The most prominent wave of these articles was based on a 2012 Stanford study[455] which generated headlines like "Organic Food 'Not Any Healthier'" (BBC), "The Organic

Fable" (*New York Times*), and "Save Your Cash? Organic Food Is Not Healthier" (*New York Daily News*). Not to be outdone, the *Daily Mail* topped it with, *"If the smug organic mob get their way, millions of families will never again be able to afford roast chicken for Sunday lunch."*

All throughout these media stories, the authors of the Stanford study claimed that there "isn't much difference between organic and conventional foods." However, their own study clearly showed that eating organic foods reduces exposure to pesticide residues and antibiotic-resistant bacteria.[456] According to their own data, only 7 percent of organic foods had pesticide residues versus 38 percent of conventional foods (besides, pesticides in conventional farming are much more toxic than the pesticides allowed in organic farming). Yet, this wasn't the only interesting finding they glossed over: their own data showed that organic foods are significantly higher in brain-boosting Omega-3 fatty acids. Finally, but perhaps not coincidentally, the Stanford authors neglected to mention that Cargill, one of the biggest conventional food producers in the world, had funded their department with more than $5 million[457] and that their statistician, Dr Ingram Olkin, had been employed by the tobacco industry to disprove the health risks of smoking.[458]

In response to the media frenzy, other researchers pointed out how their own findings contradict the Stanford study.[456,459] Considering how much *more* pesticide residues there are on conventional foods, and how much more *toxic* these are than the pesticides approved for organic farming, they estimate that eating organic foods reduces health risks from pesticide exposure by 94 percent. And these health risks, I'm sorry to say, are considerable.

Pesticides accumulate in our bodies over time and cross the

placental barrier during pregnancy. In one small study of twenty newborns in New York, every single one of them had detectable levels of multiple pesticides in their bodies.[460] Pesticides are hormone disruptors which trigger harmful epigenetic changes in foetuses and infants, and their dangers have been documented in dozens of studies. Pesticide exposure before and during pregnancy as well as in early childhood:

- Increases the risk of spontaneous abortion, birth defects, and infant death.[461-463]
- Increases the child's risk of all common childhood cancers, like leukaemia, brain and central nervous system tumours, neuroblastoma, kidney cancer, and lymphoma.[464]
- Impairs the child's brain development and intelligence.[465-467] A Californian study measured mothers' blood levels of organophosphate pesticides during pregnancy as well as their children's IQ scores by seven years of age. The children of mothers with the highest pesticide blood levels had an IQ score that was, on average, seven points lower than the children of mothers with the lowest pesticide blood levels.[466] In Europe, a comprehensive review released by the EU Parliament estimates that the reduction in children's IQ scores caused by prenatal pesticide exposure costs European countries €125 billion per year.[468]
- Increases the child's probability of attention-deficit hyperactivity disorder (ADHD), depression, and other mood disorders.[464]
- Decreases the child's lung function and increases the risk of asthma.[469-472] Another Californian study showed that a child's asthma risk roughly doubled when exposed to pesticides, and tripled when exposed to herbicides, in the first year of life.[472]

Most of these studies were based on pesticide exposure from living near conventionally farmed agricultural fields, so the exposures were almost certainly higher than you would receive from your diet. Nonetheless, according to the American Academy of Pediatrics and a whole pile of research, the main source of pesticide exposure for most children and adults *is* their diet, i.e., the pesticide residues on conventional foods.[473-477] This research also shows that switching to an organic diet for just *five days* reduces traces of pesticides in children's urine to undetectable, or nearly undetectable, levels[476] and that pesticide levels in adults' bodies can be predicted from how much organic versus conventional food they eat.[474] Consequently, a French study involving nearly 69,000 people found that, all other things being equal, eating mostly organic foods rather than conventionally farmed foods reduces your general cancer risk by 25 percent.[478]

Other "debunking organic" news stories claim that organic farms use just as many pesticides as regular farms, with the only difference being that those pesticides are of natural origin, which doesn't automatically make them safer or healthier.[479,480] There is a grain of truth to the second part of the claim but not the first. Yes, organic farms *occasionally* spray natural pesticides, and *some* of those pesticides (e.g., copper) can be quite toxic to humans or the environment. However, the most-used pesticide in organic farming is *Bacillus thuringiensis* (Bt), a naturally occurring soil bacterium which is toxic to pest insects but non-toxic to humans and other wildlife.[481,482] Compare that to the well-documented toxic effects of conventional pesticides mentioned above! As for the claim that organic farmers spray just as much pesticides as conventional ones, sorry, that's plain wrong. The rules for organic certification vary by country, but in general, organic farmers are only allowed to spray pesticides as a last resort, after ecological methods of pest control (like crop rotation, insect predators, nutrient management, mechanical weeding, physical barriers, and traps) have failed—and organic farmers have to prove this by keeping meticulous records and submitting to annual on-site inspection by organic certifiers.[483] So it's no surprise that a Greenpeace study found pesticide residues on 81 percent of conventional fruits and vegetables, but only on 13 percent of organic produce.[484] Even the "anti-organic" Stanford study supports this finding.

And what about the argument that organic farming is unsustainable, if not *immoral*, because it would be unable to feed a growing world population? "Organic debunkers" and "myth busters" like to claim that organic farming has lower yields than conventional farming.[479,480] But scientific studies comparing the yield of nearly 300 different farm crops disagree: the yields of organic farming are similar to conventional farming, up to 40 percent higher in times of drought, use 45 percent less energy, and produce 40 percent fewer carbon emissions—all while being less polluting and less harmful to wildlife.[485,486]

At the same time, advocates of genetically modified crops had promised that GMOs would increase crop yields and reduce pesticide use. This promise has been broken. In US farming, where GMOs are used extensively, pesticide use has *increased*, whereas it has declined in countries where GMOs are not permitted like France. The growth in US crop yields, meanwhile, has merely kept pace with crop yields in Europe, despite Europe not embracing GMOs.[487] Based on evidence like this, the United Nations Human Rights Council calls for "a fundamental shift towards eco-farming," stating that "scientific evidence demonstrates that agroecological methods outperform the use of chemical fertilisers in boosting food production."[488] The UN experts' message is plain and simple: the idea that pesticides are necessary to feed the world population is a myth, fuelled by the aggressive lobbying and public relations tactics of chemical companies who earn more than $50 billion per year from pesticides and fertilisers. What's more, our farming output is already sufficient to feed 9 billion people, which is 1.3 billion more than the current world population. The cause of world hunger is not insufficient farming output but a problem of food waste, poverty, and inequality.[489]

WHAT IF ORGANIC FOOD IS TOO EXPENSIVE?

It's true that organic food is more expensive—even after buying mostly organic food for a decade, I still sometimes gulp at the price difference. There are, of course, good reasons for it: organic food takes more work to produce and uses more expensive inputs. For example, animals aren't artificially fattened up with antibiotics, so they grow more slowly and don't become as big. They receive higher-quality feed, which also has to be from organic sources. They require more space, as they are raised free-range with access to land for grazing and movement. To grow organic fruits and vegetables, farmers use more labour-intensive crop rotation, hand weeding, or cover crops to control weeds. As mentioned earlier, pests are controlled with insect predators (e.g., ladybugs which eat aphids, beetles, mites, and other pests), traps, physical barriers, and with organic pesticides only being sprayed as a last resort.

Another way to think about it is this: ask not why organic food is so expensive but ask why some conventional food is so cheap. It may not be you, but someone is paying the price for the difference. It could be animals raised in appalling conditions on industrial farms, exploited farmworkers in developing countries, bees dying from pesticides, or the soil and the sea being polluted by agricultural chemicals.

Our food choices impact the world we want to leave to our kids. Insect populations are crashing on a global scale, which threatens not just human food supply but all living things that rely on them for food and pollination—a "catastrophic collapse of nature's ecosystems."[490] Moreover, we are facing climate change that will bring drought, floods, and extreme heat.[491,492] Organic farming can help us avert these disasters. Industrial agriculture and pesticide use are the main reasons for the decline in insect numbers. Thus, buying organic foods can make a difference in saving bees and other insects.[493] Likewise, a recent headline in the *Guardian* put it thusly: "Our best shot at cooling the planet might be right under our feet." Organic farming restores degraded soil, and as the soils recover, they *actively start pulling carbon dioxide from the air*. Studies estimate that a large-scale switch to organic and regenerative farming methods could offset 3–15 percent, perhaps even as much as 40 percent, of annual carbon emissions.[494,495]

If it isn't possible for you to go fully organic, the Environmental Working Group releases an annual list of the "Dirty Dozen" fruit and vegetables which are most heavily sprayed with pesticides (available at **www.growhealthybabies.com/ewg**).[496] If you just switched this produce to organic, you would already avoid the worst offenders. Here are the "Dirty Dozen," in order of the most pesticide residues to the least:

- Fruit: strawberries, apples, nectarines, peaches, grapes, and cherries.
- Vegetables: celery, spinach, tomatoes, bell/hot peppers, cherry tomatoes, and cucumbers.

According to the Centre for Science and Environment in India, you can also wash off about 75–80 percent of pesticide residues with a 2 percent salt water solution (about one teaspoon of salt per cup of water) and thoroughly rinsing in cold water.[497] Alternatively, you can wash the produce with a vinegar solution. Peeling fruits and vegetables helps as well, of course.

The Environmental Working Group also has a list of the "Clean Fifteen," the conventionally grown fruits and vegetables with the *least* amount of pesticide residues.[498] They are:

- Fruit: avocados, pineapples, mangos, papayas, kiwi, honeydew melon, grapefruit, and cantaloupe.
- Vegetables: sweet corn (though in the United States they are often GMO), cabbage, frozen sweet peas, onions, asparagus, eggplant, and cauliflower.

Another great way of accessing affordable organic food is buying from local farmers' markets. Buying directly from farmers means you don't have to pay middlemen like distributors and supermarkets, and you support local and sustainable agriculture. In our old Amsterdam neighbourhood, we had a fantastic organic farmers' market where we became members of the cooperative running the fruit and veg stand. Once every quarter, you had to help with setting up the market stall and selling the produce, and in return you permanently received a 20 percent discount on all the goods. Our food bill went down dramatically, and it helped us get to know our community and neighbours. If you live near a small, independent farm, you can also go and buy directly from them. Sometimes these farms follow organic farming methods, even if they haven't been officially certified because of the cost and hassle involved. Just ask the farmer.

We have also started growing our own vegetables on our front porch and in our tiny garden, as well as setting up growing patches in our neighbourhood's communal spaces. You'd be amazed by how much you can grow in a small area! In one experiment, a gardener grew $700 worth of produce—bell peppers, tomatoes, courgette/zucchini, lettuce, and basil—on a garden patch of just one hundred square feet (a little more than 9 m²).[499] You can also use vertical planters—hollow tubes with holes in them—to maximise your growing space. We have four of them and grow a variety of berries, vegetables, legumes, leafy greens, and herbs. It's a lot of trial and error in the beginning, but it's also great fun, especially for kids. Our daughter has loved playing with the plants since she was able to crawl. As a side benefit, it lets her grow up in touch with soil, plants, and nature, learn useful life skills, and it enriches her microbiome with plenty of beneficial soil bacteria. There is even research demonstrating that some soil bacteria have a mood-boosting, antidepressant effect by raising your serotonin levels![500-502] If you have neither a garden nor balcony space to grow vegetables, many towns and cities have community gardens that you can join.

Despite the higher cost, there is an economic argument for choosing organic food. I view it as a long-term investment in our family's health. By choosing organic, you avoid the antibiotics, antibiotic-resistant bacteria, and synthetic pesticides used in conventional farming. You also dramatically raise your intake of dietary antioxidants and Omega-3 fatty acids. Both increase the chance of staying healthy, having healthy children, and avoiding chronic illnesses. In the long run, this will save a lot of money on medication, treatments, therapies, insurance premiums, and missed work. These costs can be debilitating for families. By one estimate, having asthma in the United States costs on average more than $4,900 per year, mostly for medication and lost work time.[503] Even if your insurance covers some of it, you're still left with hundreds to thousands of dollars out of pocket. And that's not even counting how valuable health is to your quality of life. So despite the higher prices, I truly believe that organic food is worth it for your health.

CHAPTER 9

CLEANING PRODUCTS, COSMETICS, AND THEIR EFFECTS ON HEALTH

CLEANING PRODUCTS THAT POLLUTE

TV ads for cleaning products often show happy families taking deep, satisfied breaths of pine-, lemon-, or linen-scented air in their gleaming and spotless homes. What's invisible is the indoor air pollution they are inhaling. Most of the cleaning products you'll find in your supermarket aisle contain harsh and toxic chemicals like ammonia, bleach, borax, chlorides, formaldehyde, or antibacterial/antifungal compounds. These cause a laundry list of health problems like asthma, allergies, infertility, birth defects, and cancer.[504]

Of the different kinds of cleaning products, sprays are the worst for you. Researchers at the University of Cincinnati followed a group of 3,500 previously healthy individuals over nine years and tracked their cleaning habits. Those who used a spray cleaner, air freshener, or glass, furniture, and oven cleaning spray at least once a week had a 50 percent increased risk of developing asthma symptoms, and those who used three or more different types of sprays had nearly doubled their chances of being diagnosed with the disease.[505] A study conducted at the University of Bristol in the UK looked at the relationship between the use of cleaning products during pregnancy and asthma development in children. The mothers who used the most cleaning products, compared to mothers who used the least, more than doubled their children's asthma risk.[506] A long-term Norwegian study, which followed more than 6,000 people over a twenty-year period, concluded that the regular use of cleaning products at home has the same effect on lung function as smoking twenty cigarettes a day.[507]

The reason that cleaning products, and sprays in particular, can cause asthma is that they emit gasses and volatile organic compounds (VOCs) that irritate the lungs and cause inflammation of the airways. Some of the chemicals, like bleach and ammonia, can react to produce chlorine gas, which can cause asthma in a healthy person after a single high-dose exposure![504] Another issue with cleaning products are the scents and fragrances. Scents are usually mystery concoctions of dozens of undisclosed chemicals (the product label will just say "fragrance"), but unless specifically stated otherwise, they almost always include parabens and phthalates. Parabens are an antimicrobial preservative, and phthalates (pronounced "f-THA-lates") are used to make scents linger. Both disrupt the balance of hormones in your body and have been found to cause allergies, asthma, infertility, birth defects (like feminization of baby boys' genitals), and breast- and skin cancer.[508-510] The worst offenders are air fresheners—an ironic name for something which gives 20 percent of the US population headaches and breathing difficulties and which is widely considered to be the most toxic indoor air polluter.[511]

Cleaning products can also affect your health by disturbing the balance of your microbiome. Even before the coronavirus pandemic, the cleaning products industry had successfully turned us into germaphobes. Of course, in times of COVID-19, washing your hands frequently does makes sense! Any regular soap is perfectly suited for this task: It kills the coronavirus by bursting the fat membrane which holds the virus together and washes it off, along with other bacteria. But that's not enough, or so the ads for many soaps and disinfectants tell us: We need to *kill* those nasty bacteria, too, and that means buying products with antibacterial ingredients!

For decades, triclosan had been the most common antibacterial ingredient—until the US Food and Drug Administration finally banned it from household soaps and washes (but not hand sanitisers and wipes) in 2016, along with eighteen other antimicrobial chemicals. With good reason: even in low doses, triclosan harms your microbiome by decimating the population of *Lactobacilli*[512] which, as you know by now, are crucial for the developing immune system. In studies of US and Norwegian kids, the ones with the highest levels of triclosan and parabens in their body had a 50–170 percent increased risk of becoming allergic to pollen, dust, animals, and foods.[513,514] Researchers detected triclosan in nearly everyone and nearly everywhere. For example, it was found in urine samples of 75 percent of the US population as well as in 100 percent of breast milk samples in Sweden and California.[515-517]

Adding insult to injury, triclosan is utterly pointless. A review of twenty-seven different studies found that it doesn't work better than plain old soap at preventing infectious diseases and reducing bacterial levels on your hands.[518] The exact bacteria that triclosan is supposed to kill—harmful pathogens like *E. coli* and *Salmonella*—are becoming resistant to it. Steeled by their ability to resist triclosan, these bacteria are also becoming immune to other antibiotic drugs, thus adding to the health crisis of antibiotic resistance.[519]

Now that triclosan is banned from most products, can we breathe easy? I'm afraid not. The manufacturers of these antibacterial products have simply replaced triclosan and the other eighteen banned chemicals with new ones—for example, benzalkonium chloride, benzethonium chloride, and chloroxylenol. Their health effects in humans are largely unknown, but early tests in animals show that they are *more toxic* than the chemicals they are replacing.[520]

So this is the damage done to our health and the environment by the cleaning products we use on a daily basis. Their inflammatory, hormone-disrupting, microbiome-destroying chemicals combine to a toxic brew with potentially devastating effects. The New York State Department of Health looked into the relationship between birth defects and mothers' jobs during pregnancy. The highest number of birth defects were recorded for mothers who worked as cleaners or janitors. Their babies showed a significantly increased risk of being born with cleft lip or palate (a 40 percent increase), missing limbs or digits (a 140 percent increase), abnormally small or missing eyes and ears (a 170–180 percent increase), defective or missing anus or bladder (a 80–450 percent increase), and damage to the optic nerve (an almost 600 percent increase).[521] It is only a small consolation that these major birth defects are very rare and affect between 1 in 1,000 and 1 in 5,000 children, so the *absolute* risk remains small. Nonetheless, if you knew that avoiding the additional risk was possible, wouldn't you want to do it? The good news is that it's both easy and affordable to do so, and we'll talk about the how later in this chapter. But first, let's identify some other hidden chemicals lurking in your home so you can kick those out, too!

"PERSONAL CARE" PRODUCTS THAT DON'T CARE ABOUT YOUR HEALTH

Most of the chemicals—and then some—that make cleaning products so bad for our health are also in cosmetics and "personal care" products. Where else do you find antimicrobial chemicals, like the ones that have replaced triclosan? In deodorants, toothpaste, mouthwash, shaving products, creams, face powders, and colour cosmetics.[522] What about parabens, the hormone-disrupting, allergy-causing antimicrobial preservative? They are used all over the world in shampoos, conditioners, lotions, facial cleansers, and scrubs.[510] Phthalates, the fragrance carrier linked to birth defects and cancers? Banned from cosmetics in the European Union (EU) but found in nearly 75 percent of all cosmetics sold in the United States[509]—nearly all scented products. Formaldehyde, an irritant that triggers asthma, leukaemia, and various cancers?[523,524] Allowed in the United States and the EU up to supposedly "safe" limits and used mainly in water-based products as a preservative. You'll find it in body wash, lotions, sunscreen, hair gels, or nail polish.[525]

You might be wondering, if all of this stuff is so bad for us, how come it's even on sale? Surely, if you can buy it in your local supermarket or drugstore, it must have been tested and found to be safe? Unfortunately, that's not the case. In the United States, cosmetics is a $71 billion industry, and it is one of the least regulated. The US Food and Drug Administration (FDA) doesn't have the authority to require companies to do safety tests for their products, and it doesn't review or approve the vast majority of products and ingredients. Even chemicals that have clearly been linked to allergies, cancers, and major birth defects continue to be allowed if they remain below levels *thought* to be safe based on animal studies. However, as the studies described in this chapter show, there are damaging effects on health even at these supposedly "safe" levels. Nonetheless, the US cosmetics industry is allowed to police itself. As a result, cosmetics companies can use pretty much any ingredient they want, with the exception of just eleven chemicals they themselves have declared unsafe![526,527]

Things are a bit better across the border in Canada and in the EU. Canada maintains a "hotlist" of about 630 chemicals banned or restricted in cosmetics.[528] In Europe, more than 1,300 chemicals have been banned.[529] Nonetheless, many harmful ingredients like parabens and formaldehyde remain allowed in both Canada and the EU, and they are just the tip of the iceberg. A Canadian study found toxic heavy metals including lead, arsenic, and cadmium in forty-eight out of forty-nine cosmetics they tested—and none of them listed any heavy metals on the product label.[530] Generally, wherever you live in the world, it's best to limit your use of "regular" cosmetics—not just during pregnancy but forever—and switch to safer, more natural alternatives. Again, we'll get to the how later in this chapter.

"BABY CARE" PRODUCTS WITH HIDDEN NASTIES

"You want me to put WHAT on my baby?" I imagine that's what many parents would say if they knew the true ingredients of most baby products. But no matter what's in them, baby products are always marketed as "the best for your baby." Unfortunately, these marketing claims are misleading.

It's natural to assume that baby products are safe and well-tested and couldn't possibly contain chemicals that harm our little ones, but in reality, baby products are no better than cosmetics for adults. Yes, seriously. Baby shampoos, liquid soaps, and baby wipes frequently contain hormone-disrupting fragrances and parabens, as well as formaldehyde[525] or other aggressive (and aggressively unpronounceable) antimicrobials like methylisothiazolinone.[531] The latter was named "Contact Allergen of the Year 2013" by the American Contact Dermatitis Society. Cases of babies having terrible allergic reactions to wipes and other baby care products are skyrocketing.[532,533] Methylisothiazolinone might also harm brain development. Lab studies showed it to be toxic to brain cells, preventing the growth of axons and dendrites which form the connections between the neurons in the brain.[534]

Your choice of diapers is particularly important. Consider that your baby will wear one for almost twenty-four hours a day, seven days a week, for the first few years of their life—nothing else will touch your baby as much as the diaper. Your baby will absorb whatever chemicals are in there, via the skin and by breathing in the fumes and scents. Unfortunately, most big-brand diapers are terrible in this regard.

A lab test of three unnamed US big-brand diapers discovered that they all emitted chemicals in high enough levels to cause breathing problems and lung irritation in humans.[535] The chemicals included:

- Toluene, a brain-damaging solvent that gives glue sniffers their high.
- Trichloroethene, also known as "tricky" in the chemical industry. It causes nervous system depression and was used as a general anaesthetic until it was discovered to be toxic to the liver and kidneys and potentially causing permanent nerve damage as well as cancer.
- Styrene, which is toxic to the gastrointestinal tract, kidneys, lungs, and nervous system.
- Isopropylbenzene, found to cause lung and liver cancer in rats and suspected to do the same in humans.
- Ethylbenzene, which causes eye and throat irritation and dizziness and is linked to kidney and testicular cancer in rats and possibly in humans.
- Dipentene, a known skin and eye irritant.
- …and the list goes on.

Other studies have found that the dyes in coloured diapers can cause rashes and contact allergies,[536] or that diapers bleached with chlorine contain detectable levels of dioxins, a highly toxic chemical known to cause immune system damage, birth defects, and various cancers.[537,538] The World Health Organization recommends that especially pregnant and breastfeeding women should do everything they can to limit dioxin exposure to their developing foetus or baby.[539]

So what to do? The remainder of this chapter is about finding healthier, safer alternatives!

HOW TO CHOOSE BETTER CLEANING, COSMETICS, AND BABY CARE PRODUCTS

Most supermarkets and drugstores, especially the large chains, now stock a range of "natural" cleaning products, cosmetics, and baby care items. As a rule of thumb, choosing those products over the "regular" ones should be an improvement for your and your baby's health.

With that being said, descriptions like "natural," "eco," "green," "pure," "clean," "healthy," or "hypoallergenic" aren't regulated, so manufacturers can use whatever ingredients they wish and still market their products with these terms. As the market of health-conscious consumers grows, so does the temptation for manufacturers to engage in this "greenwashing." Not every cleaning product or cosmetic that calls itself green or natural is free of chemicals that can cause allergies.

For example, take Clorox, the company that introduced bleach to US households a century ago. In 2008, they were the first large consumer products company to launch a line of green cleaning products into mainstream supermarkets. This brand, Green Works, markets a range of cleaning products in green-coloured packaging splashed with a big, friendly sunflower logo. One of their products is the Green Works Naturally Derived All-Purpose Cleaner. Looking at the ingredients list,[540] what do we see?

- "Fragrance": this is usually a big red flag. According to Clorox, their fragrances are phthalate-free, but they still contain synthetic musks (hormone disruptors linked to infertility and breast cancer[541]) and literally hundreds of other chemicals[542] with unknown effects. And that's just the ones listed. Clorox says that potential allergens are not listed if their concentration is below 0.01 percent of the product.
- "Methylisothiazolinone": the neurotoxin and American Contact Dermatitis Society's "2013 Contact Allergen of the Year"

- "Liquitint Blue HP Dye and Liquitint Bright Yellow Dye": the ingredients of either are unclear (Clorox says they can be made from both synthetic and natural materials), but it seems that both of them are unnecessary for actual cleaning performance. They might be safe, but I'd still rather not have synthetic dyes in my cleaning products.

In fairness, that's a shorter list of bad stuff than you'd find on a regular cleaner, and Clorox is unusually transparent about their ingredients. Nonetheless, the Environmental Working Group's product safety rating still only gives it the grade D (with A being the best and F being the worst).[543] In their rating scale, D means "HIGH CONCERN: Likely hazards to health or the environment. May also have poor ingredient disclosure."

Or consider the case of Kimberly-Clark, another multibillion-dollar corporation, accused of greenwashing their Huggies brand of baby products. In a group of class-action lawsuits currently being heard in a California court, mothers say they were duped into buying Huggies "Pure & Natural" diapers and "Natural Care" baby wipes, believing they were safer and more eco-friendly than regular ones, but that their children developed severe contact rashes from chemicals contained in the Huggies products.[544,545] On the packaging, the "Pure & Natural" diapers (which have since been discontinued) were marketed as being made from organic cotton, but the organic cotton was only on the outside, which never touched the baby's skin anyway. On the inside, the diapers were made from the same petrochemical plastics as regular ones and contained a lotion which almost certainly had antimicrobial ingredients.[u] Huggies "Natural Care" baby wipes—still on the market and since refor-

---

u   Huggies did not disclose the ingredients, which is another major red flag.

mulated—at the time used parabens, formaldehyde-releasing chemicals, and other allergy-causing ingredients.[546]

At this point, you might be tempted to throw your hands up in frustration—do you need to do a PhD in toxicology to avoid harmful ingredients? Fortunately, there are easier ways.

The first one is to shop more from dedicated organic/eco-supermarkets, grocery stores, and health shops. Such chains exist in almost every country now, like Whole Foods (United States, Canada, UK), Planet Organic (Canada, UK[v]), Fundies and Flannery's (Australia), Alnatura and Reformhäuser (Germany), Naturalia (France), EkoPlaza (the Netherlands), Natural House (Japan), Orga Whole Foods (Korea), Nourish (in my home country, Ireland), or Life and Sunkost (in my adopted home of Norway). You can find an up-to-date list at **www.growhealthybabies.com/ecostores.**

If you don't live near such a store, try googling for "organic online stores"—these really do exist everywhere. Organic stores usually apply higher standards to the products they carry, so you are less likely to encounter greenwashed items. Whole Foods Market, for example, has comprehensive standards for cleaning products and cosmetics, both of which exclude hundreds of chemicals that are otherwise found in pseudo-green products. Cleaning products in Whole Foods' "Eco-Label Green Tier" (their highest rating) and cosmetics labelled with their "Premium Body Care Standard" are free from synthetic fragrances, formaldehyde, parabens, methylisothiazolinone, and many, many more.[547,548]

---

v   Same name in both countries but unrelated and owned by different companies.

Another way of avoiding the most harmful products is by using a free iPhone/Android app by the Environmental Working Group called EWG's Healthy Living (you can find it at **www.growhealthybabies.com/ewg**; unfortunately, the app only covers food and cosmetics sold in the United States, not cleaning products). It lets you scan the bar codes of over 120,000 items, instantly tells you the ingredients and highlights the potentially harmful ones, gives you the products' safety ratings, and shows you better alternatives. Even if you don't live in the United States, you can type in the names of cosmetics products sold internationally, and chances are pretty good you'll find them in the database.

You're probably thinking that organic, eco-, and health products are more expensive than their conventional counterparts. While that's true for organic food, in my experience it's not necessarily the case for cleaning products and cosmetics: they can even be less expensive than many well-known mass-market brands.

Lastly, you'd be surprised at how many cleaning and personal care products you can make at home using super-cheap, non-toxic, everyday ingredients. With a bit of googling, you can find simple recipes for homemade:

- All-purpose cleaners (water, vinegar, lemon juice, and some optional essential oil for scent)
- Oven cleaners and scrubbers (water, baking soda, and castile soap)
- Drain blockage removers (vinegar and baking soda)
- Air fresheners (water, alcohol, and essential oil)
- Body lotions (almond oil, coconut oil, beeswax, and essential oil)
- Body scrubs (sugar, olive oil, coffee grounds, and essential oil)

- Deodorant (coconut oil, baking soda, and essential oil)
- Hair spray (water, sugar, and essential oil)
- Hairstyling wax/putty (beeswax, coconut oil, and essential oil)
- Makeup remover (witch hazel and almond oil)
- …and many more.

So in summary, when you buy cleaning products, cosmetics, or baby care products, try to choose products free from "fragrance" and "perfume" (unless they are clearly listed as natural essential oils), parabens, phthalates, antimicrobials, and formaldehyde.[w] However, while these are the worst of the ingredients to avoid, they're not the only ones, so go for eco and natural products whenever possible. To avoid greenwashed items, shop at trustworthy eco stores that have higher standards than the large chain retailers.

---

w Formaldehyde-releasing substances are also hiding under names like quaternium-15, DMDM hydantoin, imidazolidinyl urea, diazolidinyl urea, polyoxymethylene urea, sodium hydroxymethylglycinate, bronopol, and glyoxal.

AN IMPORTANT SAFETY NOTE
ABOUT ESSENTIAL OILS

When used correctly, essential oils have powerful medicinal effects and proven therapeutic benefits. They can decrease pain, nausea, stress, and anxiety, improve moods and sleep, and have anti-inflammatory, antiviral, antifungal, and antimicrobial properties.[549-555]

Many people believe that essential oils are harmless because they are natural, widely available, and have been used for a long time. But because they are so powerful, they can also be very dangerous if misused.[556] Many essential oils can cause skin rashes, and some can be extremely poisonous when swallowed or absorbed through the skin—especially in small children.

Thus, it is extremely important to use and store essential oils safely. The US National Capital Poison Center recommends:[556]

· If an essential oil is found in a cosmetic product, use it according to label directions. Stop using it immediately if a rash or other skin reaction occurs and gently wash it off.
· If it's found in a scent, be sure that it is used and stored where children can't find it.
· If it's in a medicine, use according to label instructions ONLY.
· If you have bottles of essential oils at home, consider discarding them (safely) if you have young children. Otherwise, they MUST be locked up, out of sight and out of reach of children and pets—all the time.

To use essential oils safely and minimise the risk of allergic reactions, the Tisserand Institute recommends:[557,558]

- If you are pregnant, have a skin condition, epilepsy or asthma, are taking medications, or are in any doubt about any condition you may have, seek the advice of a doctor or suitable practitioner before using pure essential oils.
- Never put *undiluted* essential oils on your skin–this is the most common cause of allergic skin reactions.
- Never put drops of essential oil into a bath. The oils will not mix with the water but instead float on the surface as tiny undiluted droplets. These can then cling to your skin and cause allergic reactions.
- Never ingest essential oils unless advised to do so by a practitioner who is qualified/licensed to prescribe essential oils in this way.
- Don't intensively inhale essential oils (e.g., with steam inhalation) for longer than fifteen to twenty minutes.
- Limit the room diffusion of essential oils to thirty to sixty minutes, then take a break of at least thirty to sixty minutes and let in some fresh air in between.

CLEANING AND COSMETICS: WHAT WE USE

When it comes to cleaning around the house, I try to keep it simple. Remember that your goal is not to wipe out all bacteria in your environment, and that bacterial diversity is important for your baby's developing immune system.

For general-purpose cleaning (floors, wiping tables and countertops, etc.), I use a bit of castile soap—a simple, traditional soap made from vegetable oils—diluted in water. I've found Dr. Bronner's Pure-Castile Liquid Soap to be very efficient and a great value. Per bottle, it is a bit more expensive than a regular all-purpose cleaner, but I need to use a lot less. I also buy Dr. Bronner's Pure-Castile Soap Bar for hand washing. They are both widely available and score the highest safety rating from the Environmental Working Group. For other cleaning products like dishwashing liquid, dishwasher tabs, laundry detergent, and toilet cleaners, I usually buy Ecover ZERO (that's their fragrance-free line, available in Europe and the United States) or Sonett (only available in Europe so far). You can find an up-to-date list of products at **www.growhealthybabies.com/products**.

As for cosmetics, I like to use brands which only use natural and certified organic ingredients, with pure essential oils as fragrances. However, essential oils can cause skin irritations and allergic reactions in some people, so you need to find out what works for you.[x]

BABY CARE: HOW WE KEEP OUR DAUGHTER CLEAN (BUT NOT TOO CLEAN)

So what do we use to keep our daughter clean? Barely anything!

After her birth, we delayed her first bath until she was two weeks old. Babies are born covered in amniotic fluid and a white cream-like substance called vernix, which serves several important purposes. It protects a newborn baby's skin against drying out, helps regulate the body temperature, and most importantly, it has antibacterial properties. Together with amniotic fluid, vernix has been found to inhibit the growth of pathogens like Group B *Streptococcus* (the cause of blood

---

x   Especially when the essential oils have oxidised (by air contact during processing, storage, or when their container is frequently opened and closed), they contain substances which can trigger asthma attacks and skin rashes.[557,559,560] If you have pure essential oils at home, keep them refrigerated in an airtight container to prevent oxidization,[561] but also make sure to keep them away from children. See the safety note about essential oils.

poisoning, pneumonia, and meningitis), *Klebsiella pneumoniae* (another cause of pneumonia), *Listeria monocytogenes* (meningitis and other infections of the central nervous system), *E. coli* (linked to asthma and allergies), and *Candida albicans* (yeast infection linked to allergies and eczema).[316] So instead of washing off the vernix and the beneficial bacteria our daughter picked up in the birth canal (more on this in the next chapter), we let it come off her skin naturally, which takes about five to ten days.[562] When delivering your baby in a hospital, discuss with your doctor or midwife whether you can avoid washing your baby after birth. Unless there are specific reasons, there is generally no need to do so—and it actually robs your baby of a natural protective layer.

When we *did* finally give our daughter a bath, we didn't use any soap—just warm water and a soft washcloth to wipe her down gently. That's how we've been doing it until today: She gets bathed about once a week, and we only ever wash her with warm water, without soap or shampoo. Which is just as well, because like many kids, she found drinking bathwater irresistible for a while.

After a bath, we sometimes moisturised her skin with extra-virgin (unrefined) coconut oil. We also used it as a diaper balm. A big $10 tub of the good organic variety lasted us for months. The great thing about coconut oil is that it's not just a moisturiser but also has strong antimicrobial effects against pathogenic bacteria (*Listeria, Helicobacter pylori, Staphylococcus aureus,* etc.), fungi (*Candida,* etc.), and even viruses.[563,564] Because the skin of eczema sufferers is frequently infected with *Staphylococcus aureus* and *Candida* (which also causes diaper rash), studies show that it works well as a cheap and efficient eczema treatment with no side effects.[565] The antimicrobial effect comes from the lauric acid in coconut oil, which makes up about 50 percent of its contents. As an aside, guess what else is high in lauric acid? Breast milk!

As for diapers and wipes, we used brands like Naty (available worldwide), which only use fragrance-free, chlorine-free (and thus dioxin-free), and natural compostable materials like wood pulp and corn starch. They work great, too. With this simple combination—eco nappies, wipes, and coconut oil—our daughter didn't experience a single diaper rash. The baby products we used are listed at **www.growhealthybabies.com/products**.

Generally, we are quite happy to let our daughter get dirty in nature and in our garden. We encouraged her to dig around in the soil and "help" us gardening in our little fruit and vegetable patch since she could stand up on her own. As a toddler, that's when she was at her happiest! We also let her eat food that fell on the floor in our house and garden. It might take some practice to relax about this. Sometimes in my head I went, "Wait. That's so gross. Don't eat tha…Oh. Okay. Never mind. Good bacteria, good bacteria."

PART IV

BIRTH CHOICES AND POST-PREGNANCY

CHAPTER 10

HOW BIRTH CHOICES AFFECT YOUR BABY'S HEALTH

Two months after my husband and I had moved to the Netherlands, I got pregnant. When I heard that it was common for women to give birth at home there, I thought, "These people are crazy! Why would you do that? That's what hospitals are for! Give me painkillers, maybe even a C-section! There is no way, absolutely no way at all that I'll do a home birth." Nine months later, there I was—delivering our daughter in my own bedroom, without as much as having taken an aspirin. Her first contact with the outside world was landing on my husband's pillow.

Was it painful? Hell yes. Did I want to give up, go to a hospital and get an epidural, or just plain shove her back inside and try another day? You bet—but more on that in a minute. So what enabled me to push through a home birth, and what even changed my mind about it in the first place? For one, the incredible support network for pregnant women and mothers in the Netherlands—but more so, learning about the safety of various birth choices and the surprising ways in which they would affect my baby's health.

CAESAREAN VERSUS VAGINAL BIRTH

If you are like me, you might have wondered whether a C-section might be a safer, faster, and most of all, less painful way of giving birth. Some women believe it might also be less stressful for the baby. Others choose a C-section for convenience or cosmetic reasons, or they want to give birth on a date considered "lucky" in their culture.

On top of these considerations, doctors and hospitals sometimes have an incentive to push mothers towards C-sections; besides the speed and convenience, they earn the hospital more money than a vaginal delivery. The United States is the most expensive place in the world to give birth. For an uncomplicated vaginal birth, US hospitals charge an average of $32,093; for C-sections, it's the jaw-dropping amount of $51,125. Even when insurance companies cover most of these costs, families are left on the hook for thousands of dollars.[566] One US hospital even billed a mother an extra $40 fee to hold her own baby after a C-section[567]—I kid you not.

And yet, the number of C-sections has quadrupled in the last two decades, making it the most common surgical procedure performed on women of childbearing age in the world. Only 10–15 percent of pregnancies have a good medical reason for a C-section, but women and doctors choose it at much higher rates everywhere in the world, except Africa. In Asia, C-sections account for 19 percent of all births, in Europe 25 percent, in Oceania and North America around 32 percent, and in Latin America around 41 percent. In some countries, like Brazil, Egypt, or Turkey, C-section is the "new normal," with more than half of all births being delivered in this way.[568]

What surprised me was that this seemingly safe, benign, and

convenient procedure has a hidden cost that is confirmed in study after study. Children born by C-section have a 15–25 percent higher risk of getting asthma, food allergies, dust allergies, and hay fever.[569,570] The likelihood of the child developing severe mental disorders, like schizophrenia, bipolar disorder, and depression with psychosis, goes up by 13 percent.[571] Other immune problems and inflammatory conditions are also more frequently found in C-section children: type 1 diabetes, juvenile arthritis, leukaemia, inflammatory bowel disease, and general immune deficiencies.[572,573]

How could a relatively simple, one-time medical intervention have such wide-ranging consequences? The answer is that C-section babies are missing out on two crucial impulses that the immune system receives in a regular vaginal birth: first via hormones released during labour and birth, and second via the microbiome in the birth canal. In the days leading up to a natural birth, the baby's stress hormones gradually begin to rise. We tend to think of stress as a bad thing, but here, it serves an important biological purpose. In pre-labour, the mother's uterus starts contracting. This triggers the activation of the baby's hypothalamus, pituitary, and adrenal glands—the so-called HPA axis—which flood the body with stress hormones like cortisol, adrenaline, and dopamine. The HPA axis regulates moods, digestion, the immune system, and many other bodily functions. The timing of its activation is crucial and has lifelong effects on brain development, response to stress, and immune function. Scientists are calling this the HPA axis's "programming," and it happens mostly before birth. The stress hormones also speed up the maturation of the baby's organs, including the gut, during its last few days in the womb.[574,575] Then, as the baby makes its way through the birth canal in a natural birth, it is being colonised by its mother's vaginal microbiome. For some reason yet unknown, the vaginal microbiome changes just before birth, with a specific *Lactobacillus* species called *L. johnsonii* becoming highly enriched—and these microbes are particularly protective against allergies.[90]

Compare this process to a C-section. Instead of rising slowly over a few days, the baby's stress hormones surge suddenly, which changes the programming of the HPA axis. Planned C-sections are usually performed at thirty-nine weeks, so the baby is still slightly immature—and the earlier a baby is born, the higher its risk of asthma.[576] Moreover, the mother is given antibiotics in preparation for the surgery, which decimates the mother's microbiome to devastating effect (as we have explored in chapter 3 in this book). Instead of receiving a healthy vaginal microbiome from its mother, the baby is colonised by skin bacteria and the microbes in the hospital surgery room.[577,578] As a result, the microbiomes of C-section babies look very different from that of vaginally born babies. In vaginally born babies, bacteria that are crucial to modulating the baby's developing immune system—like *Lactobacilli*, *Bifidobacteria*, and *Bacteroides fragilis*—are present right from the moment of birth. In C-section babies, however, they only begin to appear between ten days to two months after birth and in lower numbers than they should. Some of these microbiome differences between C-section babies and vaginally born babies can be detected up to seven years after birth.[579,580]

In short, you should only opt for a C-section if there are medical reasons, because ensuring you have a safe birth should be the top priority. And if a C-section *does* become necessary, you can still take steps to mitigate its effects on your baby's microbiome.

The first step is to avoid being given antibiotics *before* delivery, if possible. Antibiotics are routinely administered in preparation of a C-section to avoid post-surgical uterus and wound infections, but this practice appears to be unnecessary from a medical point of view. A study at the University of Alabama showed that even in so-called high-risk mothers, antibiotics can safely be delayed until *after* cord clamping to protect your baby's budding microbiome.[581,582] Likewise, as we saw in chapter 3, taking a combination of probiotics and prebiotic fibre in the days after the C-section reduces the risk of post-surgical wound infections by more than 70 percent.[131] Discuss these options with your doctor or obstetrician in advance, and write them into your birth plan.

Second, you can try to mimic a vaginal birth with a new and relatively simple procedure called seeding. It basically involves capturing your vaginal microbiome with a swab, then gently wiping it on your baby. First, the mother is tested to ensure she has a healthy, acidic vaginal pH dominated by *Lactobacilli*, and no Strep-B or HIV infection. An hour before the C-section, a sterile, saline-soaked gauze is inserted into the vagina. Just before the surgery begins, the gauze is taken out and stored in a clean container at room temperature. Within one minute after delivery, the baby is swabbed with the gauze, starting on the lips, followed by the face, chest, arms, legs, genitals and anus, and finally the back. The swabbing only takes fifteen seconds. Early evidence suggests that it's safe and effective: babies who are seeded with this method have a microbiome more similar to vaginally born babies than to C-section babies.[583,584] However, I should note that some researchers have questioned the necessity of the procedure. In their view, the well-documented health problems resulting from C-section births are less due to the baby's lack of contact with the vaginal microbiome but more due to the use of antibiotics and the lack of labour hormones in C-sections. They also point out that there are no long-term studies yet demonstrating the safety of seeding.[585]

THE BENEFITS OF DOULAS AND BIRTH PLANS

If you are planning to have a vaginal birth, being well-prepared for the experience will calm your fears—let's face it, the prospect of squeezing a human out of your vagina is scary—and lower your odds of needing a C-section. We fear what we don't know, so information, preparation, and planning are key.

The one thing that helped me most was hearing *honest and positive* birth stories from friends who had given natural, vaginal births. They didn't glorify the experience. Some women will perceive birthing as profoundly meaningful, even beautiful, despite the pain. But many won't, and that's okay. My friends all told me that giving birth was the most painful thing they had ever endured, at least until the painkillers kicked in. But they all managed to push through. It was difficult but possible if you focused. And they told me that if they could do it, so could I.

So that was how I approached it: going into birth filled with hope and positive thoughts. As the labour progressed and got more painful, that's what I held on to. I reminded myself that the calmer I stayed, the less painful it would be, and the faster and easier my baby would find her way out. I also told myself that—as a friend had put it—my baby was the one who had to do all the work, wriggling her way through the birth canal. I just had to relax and be her guide. But more on this later: you will find my whole birth story at the end of this chapter.

Together with my husband, I also attended birth preparation classes. In the Netherlands, these are essentially free (i.e., paid for by your basic health insurance, which every citizen has), which is fantastic. Over the course of a few evenings, both parents learn about the process of birth, how to understand what's going on, and what will happen next. You practice relaxation, breathing, massage techniques, yoga and stretching positions, and how your husband or partner can help. You also review what can go wrong and how you will be helped if it happens. And you bond with the other couples who are going through the same experience.

The most important thing for me, as it turned out, was hiring a doula. A doula, sometimes also called a birth companion, is a trained professional who provides emotional and physical support to the mother during birth. Throughout most of human history, it used to be that when women gave birth, other women—mothers, grandmothers, friends—stayed by our side to cheer us on, give reassurance, share their experience, and make us feel safe and loved. But because birth has become so medicalised, that is now the exception rather than the routine. Instead, doctors, nurses, and midwives flit in and out of the hospital room to check in periodically during labour. When it comes to delivery, it's highly unusual for our mothers or friends to be there, and frequently, our husbands or partners aren't in the room either. In that situation, birth can feel like a lonely, frightening experience. Even worse, when medical staff push you towards a choice that may be against your original wishes for your birth, nobody is there to push back on your behalf.

A doula changes that. Typically, you will start meeting with your doula months before delivery. You will discuss how you imagine your dream birth and how to achieve it, as well as your fears and how to conquer them. You'll make a birth plan and build mutual trust. As soon as you go into labour, your doula will come and stay by your side until you have safely delivered the baby. Usually, a doula will also visit you in the days after birth to help you adjust to your new life as a mother. Without my doula Dana, I never would have been able to give my baby the calm, natural home birth we wanted for her.

These advantages aren't just touchy-feely but are backed up by science. Studies confirm that continuous support during birth—like the support that doulas provide—has concrete health benefits for both mother and baby. Twenty-two trials involving more than 15,000 women found that those who had continuous support were 10 percent less likely to require painkillers, 10 percent less likely to have an instrumental vaginal birth, and 22 percent less likely to have a C-section. Labour was half an hour shorter, and birth satisfaction was higher. Because the mothers stayed calmer, the babies had a better birth experience, too: they were 30 percent less likely to have a low Apgar score (a quick measure of a baby's health right after birth). This means that babies delivered with the help of doulas came into the world with a stronger heartbeat, stronger breathing, stronger arm and leg movement, and more responsive to the environment.[586]

Not every country's healthcare system is generously paying for birth preparation classes like the Netherlands does. Likewise, not everyone can afford to hire a doula—on average, their service will cost around $1,200. We were lucky in both respects. If you can afford a doula, I think it's worth every penny. It could very well end up saving you money because you're less likely to pay for expensive medical interventions. If hiring a fully qualified doula is too expensive, you can also try to find a student doula.[587] Or perhaps you have someone else—like your mother, granny, or a friend, ideally someone who has already given birth—who can stay with you during the birth. I feel that husbands and partners should be in the delivery room, too. Who would want to miss their own child being born?

Besides having birth support, planning ahead is the best way to ensure you and your baby will have the birth you want. It's a good idea to take some time to write up a one-page birth plan, which provides clear instructions to the midwives and obstetricians who will help you deliver the baby. Print them out ahead of time and have them packed in your hospital bag.

A SAMPLE BIRTH PLAN

For my birth plan, I listened to stories of friends, read birth stories online, took ideas from the birth preparation classes, and talked to my doula. Putting my wishes down on paper, including what to do if things didn't go to plan, calmed me down enormously. I felt much better prepared knowing that I had thought about and made all the important decisions in advance.

This is what my birth plan looked like, with some additional notes and explanations in parentheses:

BIRTH PLAN

Michelle and Victor Henning

We would love to have the most natural birth experience possible. It is extremely important to us to try and keep things as relaxed and natural as we can. Please keep the lights dim and the atmosphere calm.

We choose a home birth, but if that's not possible, we'd like to go to:

1st choice: Sint Lucas Andreas Hospital
2nd choice: OLVG Hospital
  (Note: These are both hospitals in Amsterdam. We researched both options and asked around regarding what the atmosphere in the delivery rooms was like and what attitudes their staff had towards natural birth.)

People present at the birth:
· My husband, Victor
· My doula, Dana Lindzon

My wishes:
· Please speak English only, as we don't speak Dutch yet.
· If we are at the hospital, no medical students attending the birth, please.
· Please don't offer me pain relief; support me in delivering naturally instead. If I do need pain relief, I will ask.
· No medical intervention without speaking to me first, please. If I can't speak for myself, please talk to my husband, Victor, or my doula, Dana.
· No continuous foetal heart monitoring unless medically nec-

essary. Please don't place a heart monitor on the baby's head in the birth canal. I would prefer the stomach monitor. I would like to keep as mobile as possible during the birth; is there an option of wireless monitoring?

- No episiotomy.

  (Note: An episiotomy is a surgical cut between the vagina and the anus made just before delivery to avoid tearing the perineum. It's still routine in many places, but evidence shows that it has higher infection rates and takes longer to heal than a natural tear.[588] The World Health Organization now advises against routine episiotomies.)

- Please don't wash the baby after delivery. Please pass her to me immediately and place her on my skin.

  (Note: This was to ensure that our baby could keep the vernix on her skin, which has several important functions and health benefits. See also "Baby Care: How We Keep Our Daughter Clean (But Not Too Clean)" in chapter 9 for more details.)

- Please delay the cord clamping until the pulsing stops. My husband, Victor, would like to feel the pulsing.

  (Note: In many places, it's standard practice to clamp the umbilical cord immediately after birth–it was thought that this would reduce jaundice. Instead, it means that the baby loses out on valuable blood it would otherwise receive. A Swedish study found that babies whose cord clamping was delayed by at least three minutes had 45 percent more blood iron and a 90 percent lower risk of iron deficiency. In a follow-up study four years later, these children also had more advanced brain development with better social and fine motor skills.[589,590] A good supply of iron is crucial for healthy immune and brain development, as you saw in chapter 7.)

- If I need a C-section for any reason, please help me to have the gentlest one I can. Please keep the lights as low as possible and place the baby on my chest as soon as possible. I would like to keep her with me at least for the first hour and to breastfeed and bond with her skin to skin as soon as I can. I want my husband with me at all times.

· After delivery, I or my husband have to be with the baby at all times.

· Please do not give the baby any medications (not even paracetamol) without checking with us first.

COULD A HOME BIRTH BE RIGHT FOR YOU?

Throughout most of human history, women have given birth in their own home, but as access to hospitals improved during the twentieth century, home births have become extremely unusual. The rate of planned home births ranges from 0.1 percent in Sweden, to 1–2 percent in the United States and UK, to about 20 percent in the Netherlands.[591] I most likely would never have considered the option had I not coincidentally lived in Amsterdam when I got pregnant. As I said at the beginning of this chapter, before I learned more about home births, they seemed scary, irresponsible, and even crazy!

To my big surprise, medical studies say otherwise. If you have no known pregnancy complications, as well as a hospital close by in case of emergencies, it turns out that planned home births are just as safe for the baby and *safer* for the mother. Mothers who choose a home birth have lower rates of postpartum bleeding, perineal tearing, and lower rates of medical interventions such as episiotomy, instrumental vaginal birth, and C-section. They also are much happier with the birthing experience due to the more relaxed environment of their own home and feeling more in control of the experience.[652]

Support for home births is coming from unexpected places. In the UK, the Royal College of Obstetricians and Gynaecologists and the Royal College of Midwives have issued a joint statement promoting their advantages:[592] "There is no reason why home birth should not be offered to women at low risk of complications, and it may confer considerable benefits for them and their families. There is ample evidence showing that labouring at home increases a woman's likelihood of a birth that is both satisfying and safe, with implications for her health and that of her baby."

So if you are having a healthy pregnancy, and there is good support for home births where you live—midwife support, regular checkups to make sure that you have no known complications, access to hospitals nearby—I would encourage you to consider it. I'm not going to lie: my home birth was painful and scary at times. I cursed and wished I was in a hospital being pumped full of painkillers more than once. But with the support of my doula and my husband, I found a way of overcoming the fear and pain, and it enabled me to give my daughter the gentle, natural birth I had dreamed of.

MY BIRTH STORY

I had been in early labour for a few days, running up and down the stairs, bouncing on a gym ball, eating spicy Korean food—trying everything to encourage our daughter to make her way out. I was 3 cm dilated, yet there was still no sign of her coming. So at forty-one weeks and three days, we decided to let the midwife break my waters. We thought I had a good chance of going into full labour and avoiding a hospital induction. Our dream was to give our baby a gentle entry into the world in our own home. I desperately wanted to avoid hospital interventions and exposing her to pain-relief drugs. My doula supported me in this goal, yet had also cautioned me that labour pain was a pain unlike anything I had ever experienced before. I thought, "How bad could it be?"

The midwife broke my waters at 11:30 a.m., then left my home to see other patients. The contractions started almost immediately after. They were fast and furious and coming only five minutes apart, with agonizing pain in between. It was quite overwhelming. Gone were all my well-intentioned plans of slowly easing into labour with time for relaxation, warm showers, and baking snacks to keep myself busy. My husband called my doula, Dana, to tell her my contractions had started. I was still convinced that the pain would ease soon, and I would get those breaks between contractions that people had been telling me about. So I told Dana that I was fine for now and she didn't need to hurry. I was wrong. Within fifteen minutes, I was crying out for Dana to come.

She arrived soon after. For an hour, we tried different positions and sitting on a gym ball, but the pain wasn't letting up. I wasn't getting any breaks at all from the pain in between the contractions. We had prepared for a water birth with an inflatable birthing pool in our bedroom, so we decided to fill it up to try to provide me with some relief. I was really struggling at this point—I wanted to give up and get pain medication. I began begging my husband to bring me to the hospital. I told him I couldn't go on anymore, that I couldn't take any more pain.

Knowing that this was not what I really wanted in my heart and that my dream was to have my daughter at home, my husband and my doula hatched a plan to get me through. My doula started to sing a beautiful song about birth, and within moments, I started to sing along. Something changed. I got into the pool and continued to sing. With my eyes closed and mind focused, I started to make up songs for my daughter. I sang through each wave of pain that washed over me. I swayed in the water and visualised my body opening. I imagined I was singing directly to my daughter, letting her and my body know it was all okay. I kept focusing on the thought that every bit of pain meant I was getting closer to meeting her and holding her in my arms.

When my midwife returned, my concentration was broken. I started panicking again, asking for the hospital, and thinking I couldn't cope with the pain. But my midwife also encouraged me to stay at home, telling me that if I had managed without pain relief so far, I would be able to see it through. After a few minutes, I found my focus and my voice again. I sang for the next four hours straight, changing the words with each transition of the labour. Singing not only released endorphins but kept my breathing flowing. I felt that if I could keep my body loose and my baby calm, things would keep moving, and we could achieve the beautiful birth I had wanted. Stress was only going to slow the labour down.

Meanwhile, the sun had set, and it had gone dark outside. The lights in my bedroom were dimmed to a soft orange glow, and I was surrounded by my midwife, my doula, my husband, and a good friend who had also joined us. I continued to sing through the pain until over 9 cm dilation. My husband stayed with me the whole time, rubbing my shoulders. He didn't leave my side for the whole eleven hours of labour.

Finally, after fifty-nine minutes of pushing, our daughter arrived—landing on my husband's pillow. Accompanied on her way out by the sound of my singing, she had stayed calm during birth, with a steady heart rate. Now she was snugly nestled in my arms and feeding on my breast. It was the most incredible moment of my life.

There is nothing easy about the pain of birth, but it can be conquered. I'm thankful that I had the opportunity to give birth at home in our own bedroom. We don't live in the same house anymore, but I have a photo of the spot where my daughter was born. I still look at it sometimes and smile.

BREASTFEEDING: A BOOST FOR YOUR BABY'S HEALTH

Breast milk is a marvel, finely tuned over millions of years of evolution. In fact, based on hundreds of medical studies, breastfeeding is one of the best gifts you can give to your child for their long-term health and development.[593] That is why the World Health Organization recommends exclusive breastfeeding for at least six months and supplemental breastfeeding until age two.[594] Breastfeeding helps babies' sensory and cognitive development, protects them against infectious and chronic diseases, reduces their risk of dying due to common childhood illnesses, and has many other long-term psychological and neurological benefits.

How does breast milk accomplish these wonders? For starters, it contains an optimal and complete mix of nutrients—essential fatty acids and amino acids, carbs, proteins, vitamins, minerals, and more. Babies need literally *nothing* else to eat or drink for the first few months of life, not even water (in fact, giving water to babies is harmful![y]). The composition of breast milk is always changing and is highly tailored to the needs of the individual child—for example, breast milk for baby boys has more fat and protein, while breast milk for baby girls has more calcium.[595] Breast milk produced during the day stimulates the baby and makes it more active, while breast milk produced in the evening makes the baby sleepy by releasing more relaxation hormones like melatonin and GABA.[596,597] Want to raise the melatonin levels in your breast milk even further? Watch a comedy! A Japanese study had one group of mothers watch the Charlie Chaplin movie *Modern Times*, while a control group watched a decidedly not-funny program with weather information. The breast milk melatonin levels of mothers who had seen the comedy were elevated by 34 percent, whereas it stayed the same in mothers subjected to the weather information. Even more amazing: in mothers who had eczema, the comedy nearly doubled their breast milk melatonin levels, which led to decreased allergic responses in their babies![598]

One of the least known, but most important, functions of breastfeeding is to keep sharing the mother's immune system with the newborn baby. Once babies leave the safety of the womb, they aren't just exposed to the friendly microbes we have been talking about in this book but also to dangerous bugs and viruses—while their immune systems aren't fully developed yet. By relying on their mother's immune system shared through breast milk, babies can save precious energy fighting off infections and focus on growing instead. This shared immune system protects the baby in at least four ways that we know of:

---

y   By filling a baby's belly with water, it causes them to miss out on vital nutrients from breast milk or formula. If you give a baby too much water, it can make the sodium levels in their blood drop rapidly, and they can get seriously ill.

1. Breast milk is rich in antibodies, cytokines, and lauric acid, which prevent the growth of harmful microbes and fungi. Baby saliva also contains substances that react with breast milk to form hydrogen peroxide—yep, bleach!—which can kill bad bacteria like *Staphylococcus aureus* and *Salmonella*.[599] This is called passive immunity.

2. Breast milk lets the mother's immune system share its knowledge with the baby's immune system. The breast milk contains immune cells targeting specific threats, and the baby's body makes copies of these immune cells. The researchers who discovered this process termed it "maternal educational immunity," because the baby's immune system learns from the immune information provided by the mother.[600] This discovery could help improve vaccinations: some vaccines—like the one against tuberculosis—are either not safe or not very effective for newborns. Instead, the vaccine could be given to the mother, who would then transfer her immunity to the baby.[601]

3. Breast milk contains a "SWAT Team" of immune cells called innate lymphoid cells (ILCs). This SWAT team serves multiple functions: they direct white blood cells (which make up the largest cell population in breast milk) to gobble up invading viruses and bacteria, they regulate the baby's budding microbiome by telling its immune system *not* to attack friendly bacteria, and they help form the protective lining of the baby's gut.[602–604]

4. Perhaps most amazingly, breastfeeding provides a feedback loop between your baby's immune system and yours—it lets your baby call your body for help in fighting the bugs they are dealing with at any given moment. During breastfeeding, any infectious bugs that a baby might have caught are transferred from the baby's mouth onto the mother's breast, where they enter through the areola and nipple. An

immune system inside the breast, called the enteromammary immune system, starts producing the right antibodies to fight the infection and passes them back to the baby via the breast milk.[605,606]

Thanks to this function as your baby's on-call immune system, exclusive breastfeeding for at least four to six months can save lives. It reduces the risk of serious stomach and lung infections by about 50 percent. These infections are the most common causes of hospitalisation and death in newborns, and accordingly, exclusive breastfeeding for four to six months cuts the risk of infant hospitalisation and death in half![607-609] Breastfeeding is such an important safety net to a newborn's health that initiating it within the first *hour* after birth can significantly reduce the baby's risk of death in the first month. A large World Health Organization study in Ghana, India, and Tanzania involving nearly 100,000 babies found that neonatal mortality was much lower if breastfeeding began in the first hour of life (11 deaths per 1,000 births), compared to later within the first twenty-four hours (15 deaths per 1,000 births) or between day one to four of life (17 deaths per 1,000 births).[610]

In addition to preventing acute illnesses and medical emergencies, breastfeeding also reduces the risk of milder infections, like tummy bugs and ear infections, by 50 percent,[608,611] and it protects babies against chronic diseases. Breast milk is literally a "living" fluid. It contains over 700 different strains of beneficial bacteria and the very specific prebiotic fibres (oligosaccharides) needed to feed them. The composition of these beneficial bacteria changes over the first six months of breastfeeding, which suggests that different kinds of microbes might be important for the baby's health at different stages of development.[40] Breast milk is the primary way of giving your baby a healthy microbiome,[612] which as we saw in previous chapters, is key to establishing a balanced immune system and avoiding inflammatory and atopic diseases.

Medical researchers all over the world have investigated whether breastfeeding can prevent asthma, eczema, and allergies. The answer, based on studies done in Australia, Canada, Finland, Germany, the Netherlands, Qatar, Sweden, the United States, and elsewhere, is a resounding YES. Overall, they find that exclusive breastfeeding for at least three to four months lowers the risk of these atopic diseases by around 30–40 percent and even more if there is a family history of atopy.[613-622] These benefits appear to be lasting for life. For example, researchers at the University of Helsinki Children's Hospital tracked the health of 150 children until the age of seventeen. Of the children who had been breastfed for only a month or less, 23 percent had an atopic disease by age one, increasing to a staggering 65 percent by age seventeen. By comparison, of the children who had been breastfed for six months or longer, only 11 percent had an atopic disease by age one and 42 percent by age seventeen.[620]

Unsurprisingly, breastfeeding also helps to prevent other chronic diseases, especially inflammatory conditions of the gut and digestive system. As we discussed in chapter 2, a healthy microbiome lowers inflammation in the entire digestive tract and strengthens the gut wall. This is what breast milk does via beneficial microbes as well as other bioactive compounds.[603,622] Breastfed children are just half as likely to suffer from painful inflammatory bowel diseases like ulcerative colitis and Crohn's disease later in life.[623] If the baby is still being breastfed when gluten is first introduced into the baby's diet, the risk of celiac disease is cut in half.[611] Further, because the microbiome modulates our insulin resistance and how we store fat, breastfed children are 10–20 percent less likely to become obese, and 20–40 percent less likely to become diabetic later in life.[611,624,625]

Breastfeeding protects children against life-threatening illnesses, too. I think that for us parents, few things are scarier than the idea of our little ones getting cancer. Breastfeeding dramatically reduces children's cancer risk, as dozens of medical studies have concluded. For example, a team of Israeli doctors surveyed twenty-five different studies going back to 1960 to examine the effect of breastfeeding on leukaemia, the most common childhood cancer. Their finding: breastfeeding for six months or longer reduces the risk of leukaemia by 20 percent. In other words, nearly twenty out of one hundred cases of childhood leukaemia could be prevented simply by breastfeeding.[626] British researchers discovered a similar protective effect against Hodgkin's lymphoma, a cancer of the lymphatic system, and neuroblastoma (nerve cell cancer), the third most common childhood cancer. Breastfeeding reduces the risk of these cancers by about 25 percent and 40 percent, respectively.[627] One of the reasons is that a certain chemical called Alpha1H, which only occurs in breast milk, helps to break up and dissolve tumours in the body. Alpha1H is so effective at killing tumours that scientists are now racing to turn it into an anti-cancer drug more effective than chemotherapy but without the nasty side effects.[628]

But those are "just" the benefits of breastfeeding for preventing chronic and life-threatening illnesses. The advantages go further still. Several studies have found that breastfeeding increases children's intelligence, resulting in potentially better grades in school and perhaps even higher education and salaries in adulthood.[611,629] A smaller but no less tangible long-term advantage of breastfeeding is that it makes children less picky eaters later.

This will reduce the number of times you bang your head on the table in frustration during meals. Formula always tastes the same, somewhat bland and sweet, while breast milk changes its flavour based on your diet. The more varied your diet, the more your baby gets used to these flavours. A study of nearly 14,000 children in Belarus showed that exclusive breastfeeding for three months halved problematic eating behaviours at age twelve.[358,630]

Breastfeeding also releases hormones, especially oxytocin and prolactin, which are good for both you and your baby. Oxytocin is sometimes called the "love hormone"; it plays a central role in all human connections that we form. Our levels of oxytocin rise when we touch, hug, or kiss a loved one. It increases feelings of trust and warmth, and it's a very potent anti-stress, antidepressant, and anti-inflammatory hormone. That's why breastfeeding has been found to:[631-634]

- Strengthen the lasting bond between mother and baby.
- Lower mothers' stress levels and improve their moods.
- Reduce the risk of postpartum depression.
- Increase mothers' overall mental and physical health.

A few more things you will appreciate: Breastfeeding is cheaper than formula. You don't have to buy the formula, bottles and teats, or sterilising equipment. It's also a lot easier, once you get the hang of it (more on that in a minute). Instead of getting up in the middle of the night and stumbling into the kitchen to boil water, sterilise bottles, scoop powder, and mix formula, you just stay in bed and whip out your boob. On average, mothers who breastfeed exclusively get thirty minutes more sleep every night.[635] Considering how sleep-deprived we mothers are, that makes a hell of a lot of difference.

In the medical journal *The Lancet*, researcher Keith Hansen argues, "If breastfeeding did not already exist, someone who invented it today would deserve a dual Nobel Prize in medicine and economics." Hansen estimates that on a global scale, increased breastfeeding could save 820,000 lives and add $302 billion to the world economy per year.[636] Formula companies, however, would very much like you to believe that there is no difference between breast milk and formula.

Just consider: infant formula is a global $50 billion industry, and breastfeeding is their primary competitor. So formula companies subtly undermine breastfeeding by pretending to support it—by producing leaflets with "helpful" breastfeeding tips and guidelines that make breastfeeding sound uncomfortable, impractical, painful, or embarrassing.[637,638] These leaflets—along with free formula samples—are then distributed through hospitals and doctor's practices. This gives both the leaflets and formula samples the sheen of being "endorsed" by medical professionals. A study at the University of Rochester in New York showed that women who had received the formula company materials were *six times* more likely to stop breastfeeding soon after birth.[639] Another study in Oregon reached the same conclusion: most American mothers receive free formula as "gifts" in their hospital discharge packs (in the UK, this is illegal!), and as a result, they are much more likely to stop exclusive breastfeeding soon after birth.[640]

In developing countries, the formula companies' tactics are even more brazen. Investigative reporters uncovered how three of the largest formula producers—Nestlé, Abbott, and Mead Johnson—were "earning the loyalty" of doctors and nurses in the Philippines with "free trips to lavish conferences, meals, tickets to shows and the cinema, and even gambling chips." Unfortunately, these tactics are paying off. Some of the poorest mothers in these countries are starving themselves so they can afford to buy formula, which they believe is better for their babies than their own breast milk, thanks to the formula companies' marketing.[641]

GETTING HELP WITH BREASTFEEDING

Breastfeeding is supposed to be the most natural thing in the world, and yet it can be surprisingly difficult to get started. I should know—it took me five weeks to get our daughter to latch on to my breast properly. It was painful, stressful, frustrating, and demoralizing, and if I hadn't known about the far-reaching health benefits of breastfeeding, I might have given up. In the end, we only succeeded because we got help.

We started noticing problems soon after our daughter's birth. Even though she tried to latch on to my breast, she didn't seem to succeed for very long. Her weight started dropping, and we began to panic.

In the Netherlands, every new mother is provided with home care by a maternity nurse, the Kraamzorg, for eight to ten days after birth. The nurse comes to your home every day, helps you look after the baby, and makes sure you are recovering from birth. They even help clean your home and sometimes cook for you. The Kraamzorg is covered by your basic health insurance, so you don't have to pay for this brilliant service.

As much as we appreciated the Kraamzorg service, unfortunately our particular maternity nurse was of no help with our breastfeeding problem. On the contrary, the more our daughter's weight dropped, the more the nurse pressured us to give up on breastfeeding and feed formula instead. The nurse even threatened that if we couldn't stop the weight loss, our daughter would be taken to a hospital and fed formula there. We were desperate but didn't want to give up trying yet. So I pumped breast milk day and night, and Victor fed our daughter the breast milk with little spurts from a syringe. Each feeding took hours. Fortunately, this stopped her weight loss, and after a week, she started to slowly gain weight again.

Still, she struggled with latching on to the boob, so we turned to La Leche League (LLL) for help. It sounds like a superhero organisation, and to me, that's what it is! LLL is a global non-profit organisation dedicated to helping mothers breastfeed. There's probably a local LLL group near you! We had attended a breastfeeding course at our local Amsterdam LLL group before birth and hoped the breastfeeding teacher there, Gina, could help us. While Gina was wonderfully supportive and gave lots of tips and advice, none of it was a silver bullet; after two weeks of trying, our daughter still couldn't latch, and whenever she was on my boob, it was really painful, which it shouldn't have been.

Gina suggested a contact of hers, a nurse who was a certified "lactation consultant," meaning she had special training in solving breastfeeding problems. She came to our home and quickly diagnosed our daughter with ankyloglossia, more commonly known as tongue-tie (it turns out that Victor has it, too). In babies with tongue-tie, the membrane that connects the underside of the tongue to the floor of the mouth is unusually short and thick, which can restrict the tongue's movement. It's not that uncommon—around 5–10 percent of babies have it, and it can lead to breastfeeding problems and painful breastfeeding.[642,643] The lactation consultant performed a quick surgery called frenectomy on our daughter, which cuts the small membrane under the tongue. Frenectomy removes the restriction on the tongue's movement, heals quickly, and has no known side effects.[643] It seemed fairly painless, too—our daughter cried briefly but was okay again shortly after, without needing any painkillers.

Unfortunately, the frenectomy did not solve our breastfeeding problem either. It made it slightly less painful, but another week having passed, our daughter still had problems latching on to the boob. The lactation consultant was stumped—there seemed to be no medical reason why breastfeeding was such a struggle. By now, it had been a month since our daughter's birth, and we were still supplementing her breastfeeding with pumped breast milk in bottles. The lactation consultant thought there was nothing else we could do—just wait for her to get bigger, which would hopefully make latching easier.

We decided to look for help elsewhere. I asked my doula, Dana, for the best person she knew, and she recommended another lactation consultant, Myrte van Lonkhuijsen. You could hardly find somebody more experienced: Myrte had been the chairwoman of the Dutch Association of Lactation Consultants for five years. I reached out to her. The same afternoon, Myrte came cycling to our house on her old Dutch bike, a big professional baby weighing scale strapped onto the rear carrier. She radiated calm, confidence, and kindness, combined with an absolute determination to fix this problem. I loved her immediately! And what happened next felt like pure magic.

She made me show her our attempt at breastfeeding and how our daughter tried to latch. She looked at it for a minute, then said, "Ah, I've seen this before. Let's try something." She made me point my index finger, gently guided it to about an inch under my nipple, at the outer edge of my areola, with my finger pointing slightly upwards. Then she told me to press a bit inwards and upwards, which made the nipple point a bit downwards. Myrte has a funny name for it. She calls it the Concorde method, because the nipple angles down like the nose of the supersonic Concorde passenger plane did for takeoff and landing.

You can find the full manual with illustrations of the Concorde method on Myrte's website (via **www.growhealthybabies.com/concorde**). Here's a snippet:

A baby with a tongue-tie or receding chin may benefit from a slightly different way to offer your breast. The aim is to get from a pinched nipple to a nice wide grasp.

The Concorde is a way of latching the baby to the breast in order to have a comfortable and effective feed for both of you. Why Concorde? Because you get to angle your nipple like this:

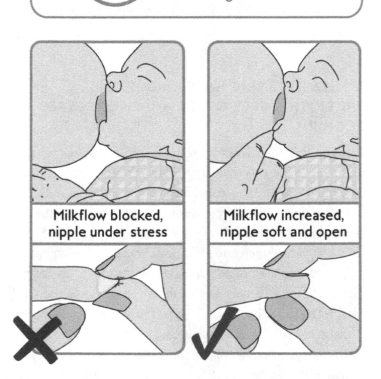

Milkflow blocked, nipple under stress

Milkflow increased, nipple soft and open

Myrte's method made it possible for our daughter to get the whole nipple into her mouth. It worked like a miracle. Barely fifteen minutes after Myrte had stepped into our door, our daughter was happily and painlessly latched on to my boob and drinking away. It was the beginning of her lasting love affair with boobie, and we stopped needing to pump breast milk that same afternoon. Myrte has since helped a few of my friends solve their breastfeeding problems, sometimes even via Skype.

So you see, I struggled, I cried, I despaired, and I needed lots of help and weeks of trying until I was able to breastfeed successfully. If you want to breastfeed but are struggling, please don't give up hope. Get help as soon as you can and keep trying. It's worth it!

IF BREASTFEEDING ISN'T AN OPTION: PROBIOTICS, PREBIOTICS, AND HYDROLYSED FORMULA

Perhaps your job makes it impossible to breastfeed, or there are medical reasons that prevent you from doing so. In that case, one possibility to consider is donated breast milk from a human milk bank. Perhaps you find the idea of giving your baby another woman's breast milk strange, but donor breast milk is rigorously screened and pasteurised, so it is completely safe. However, it is also extremely scarce, so it is mostly reserved for sick, hospitalised newborn babies.[644] In any case, the World Health Organization, UNICEF, and the American Academy of Pediatrics (AAP) all recommend that donor human milk should be the first alternative over formula when maternal milk is not available, particularly for babies born prematurely.[645]

If neither breastfeeding nor donor breast milk is an option, you can nonetheless make formula choices that boost your baby's chances of good health. It's crucial that the formula you choose contains both added DHA and ARA (the fatty acids we discussed in chapter 5). Both of these are vitally important to your baby's brain development, and studies show optimal effects when the ratio of DHA to ARA is between 1:1 (i.e., equal amounts of DHA and ARA) and 1:1.5 (slightly more ARA than DHA, similar to breast milk).[646]

Next, I would suggest choosing formula that contains both probiotics and prebiotic fibre—or you can mix some into the formula yourself. As you saw in the "Probiotics" section of chapter 7, there is good evidence that giving your baby probiotics from birth can strongly reduce its risk of asthma, eczema, and allergies. The most effective probiotic bacteria are *Lactobacillus rhamnosus*, *Lactobacillus paracasei*, *Bifidobacterium longum*, *Bifidobacterium lactis*, and *Bifidobacterium breve*.

Likewise, prebiotic fibre has strong protective effects against atopic diseases by fostering the growth of a healthy microbiome. In one trial at the University of Milan, formula-fed babies who received a mix of prebiotics (galacto-oligosaccharides and fructo-oligosaccharides, about one tablespoon per litre of formula during the first six months of life) had a 50 percent lower rate of eczema, a 66 percent lower rate of asthma, and an 85 percent lower rate of allergic skin reactions than formula-fed babies who were given a placebo.[201] Another trial in the Ukraine found a similar reduction in asthma risk and a 72 percent reduction in food allergies.[179] In other studies, the results weren't as clear-cut but pointed in the same direction: prebiotics reduce the risk of eczema and allergies in formula-fed babies.[647-650] You can find prebiotics that are suitable for babies in most health shops. Just make sure to monitor how your baby reacts to them—if the dose is too high (generally, above 20 g/day), they can cause bloating, tummy discomfort, and diarrhoea.[651,652]

Another effective allergy prevention strategy is choosing so-called hydrolysed formula instead of regular formula. In hydrolysed formula, the cow's milk protein has already been broken down, either partially or fully. For preventing allergies, both varieties—partially or fully hydrolysed—appear to be equally effective.[653] A recent meta-analysis that combined the results of eight medical trials found that babies who received hydrolysed whey formula, instead of regular cow's milk formula, were around 37–38 percent less likely to develop eczema and allergies.[654] You should be able to find both partially and fully hydrolysed (sometimes also called extensively hydrolysed or hypoallergenic) formula in regular shops and supermarkets—though in some countries, including the UK, fully hydrolysed formula is only available by prescription.

Another popular alternative to cow's milk formula is soy-based formula; it accounts for about 25 percent of all formula sold in the United States. However, my recommendation would be to avoid soy formula. Let me explain why. Soy formula is marketed as an option for children who already have cow's milk allergy and is sometimes portrayed as being helpful in preventing allergies. However, it is not particularly suitable in either case: many children who have cow's milk allergy also have a soy allergy, so hydrolysed formula is the better choice.[655] As for preventing allergies, soy formulas aren't any better than cow's milk formulas—in fact, they are probably worse. The data suggests that soy formula actually increases your child's allergy risk.[656] Besides, like all soy-based foods and drinks, they contain plant oestrogens which can mimic the effects of oestrogen, the female sex hormone, in the body. Studies demonstrate that high exposure to plant oestrogens can cause an early onset of puberty and increased breast cancer risk in girls, as well as reduced fertility in boys. In rare cases, if the plant oestrogen exposure is high in the womb, birth defects in the baby's genitals can occur.[657,658]

A few studies have investigated whether soy formula-fed children suffer from any ill health effects later in life. One found that 17 percent of adults who had been fed soy formula suffered from asthma or allergies versus only 10 percent of adults who had been fed cow's milk formula. Moreover, women suffered from longer and more painful periods if they had been fed soy formula.[659,660] Two other studies discovered that in babies who already suffer from inadequate thyroid hormone production, soy formula makes the problem worse.[655] Hence, I would not choose soy formula.

Last but not least, choose organic formula if possible and pay attention to the amount of added sugar—the less sugar, the better!

WEANING AND INTRODUCING SOLID FOODS

Medical researchers have long suspected that the timing of when solid foods are introduced to a baby's diet could influence the development of allergies. The recommendations and guidelines on when to introduce solids are currently shifting based on new research.

In the 1960s, parents introduced solids to their babies' diets when they were, on average, about two months old. In the 1970s, based on the suspicion that the early introduction of gluten could be behind the rise in celiac disease, guidelines started recommending delaying solid foods until after four months. By the late 1990s, guidelines were changed again to recommend delaying solids until after six months. This is still the World Health Organization's position: it recommends exclusive breastfeeding for six months, then introducing solids, and—crucially—continued breastfeeding until two years of age.[661]

Recently, new medical trials have suggested that delaying the introduction of solids beyond six months might in fact *increase* the allergy risk. According to these trials, there is a "window of opportunity" between the age of four to six months for introducing solid foods. Introducing solids, especially allergenic foods like egg, nuts, and dairy, outside this window of opportunity—both earlier *or* later—could increase the risk of developing allergies.[653,662] Another view is that the *overlap* of breastfeeding with the introduction of solids is the key to allergy prevention, because the immune-regulating compounds in breast milk reduce the likelihood of allergic reactions to the food being introduced.[663,664]

As discussed in chapter 4, introducing yoghurt with live probiotic bacteria to your child's diet early is another proven eczema and allergy prevention strategy. Three studies in Switzerland, Japan, and New Zealand found that children who regularly consumed yoghurt in their first year of life had a 30–70 percent lower risk of eczema and a 40–85 percent reduced risk of allergies.[186-188] The more often a child eats yoghurt, the greater the risk reduction—ideally, it should be at least once a week. Make sure that the yoghurt is full-fat, unsweetened, unpasteurised, and contains live bacteria, or make your own yoghurt at home!

Altogether, the guidelines for introducing solids are as follows:

- Before you introduce solids, your baby has to be able to sit up without support and have sufficient control of his/her neck and head.

- Keep breastfeeding *throughout* the period of introducing solids—at least until six months of age but ideally longer. To me, this is crucial: the idea is to give your baby an initial taste of the foods and let its immune system get acquainted with them *while breastfeeding*, and not to replace breastfeeding with solids.
- Starting between four to six months of age, first introduce non-allergenic foods like fruit, vegetables, rice, oats, and—given its proven allergy prevention benefits—yoghurt. Introduce them as single ingredients, not mixed up, and don't go too fast—leave a few days before introducing each new food.
- Acidic foods like berries, citrus fruits, and tomatoes can cause minor skin rashes or hives around the mouth—don't panic if they do. This is typically just a local skin irritation from the acids and histamine-releasing compounds in these fruits, not a full-blown allergic reaction. However, if in any doubt, contact your doctor to discuss.
- Once you have successfully introduced some non-allergenic foods and your baby tolerates them well, start introducing allergenic foods like dairy, eggs, nuts, wheat/grains, and seafood. When introducing the allergenic foods, give your baby a tiny taste first and see if there is any reaction. Wait at least a few hours before giving more. If there is no allergic reaction, you can gradually increase the amount of food over the next few days. If there is still no reaction after three to five days, you can move on to introducing the next allergenic food. Do it *at home*, not in a restaurant and day care. To be on the safe side, I'd suggest doing it on a weekday when doctors and pharmacies are open.
- As you may recall from our discussion of probiotic sup-

plements, recent medical trials demonstrated that giving children *Lactobacillus rhamnosus* probiotics alongside increasing doses of allergenic foods prevented, and even reversed, allergic reactions. Based on these findings, consider giving your baby a daily dose of probiotics containing *L. rhamnosus* while introducing solids and especially allergenic solids. You can find links to supplements at **www.growhealthybabies.com/supplements**.

- If your baby already has signs of allergies, eczema, or asthma, see a doctor specialised in allergies (called an allergist) to create a personalised plan for introducing solids.
- Lastly, use home-cooked weaning foods and avoid commercial foods. As with formula, manufacturers make these too sweet to ensure that babies will gobble them up with little resistance—thus instilling unhealthy flavour preferences and a "sweet tooth" in your baby.[665]

SUMMARY

BRINGING IT ALL TOGETHER

Protecting your child from asthma, eczema, and allergies is not just down to the genetic lottery or pure luck. You have the power to dramatically improve your child's chances of being healthy by making choices that promote your health and well-being. I hope that you have gained some new insights and ideas from this book and that perhaps you have been inspired to make some changes to your lifestyle.

But "with great power comes great responsibility," and this responsibility can also be a burden. It's hard enough to grow a human being inside you and to look after two bodies instead of just one, even if you don't have to suddenly adopt new habits. I was fortunate: my husband and I hadn't been dealt the best cards in terms of health, but thanks to my training as a nutritional therapist, we were already leading a pretty healthy lifestyle. I didn't need to change all that much when I became pregnant.

Even so, as we started doing the research for this book, I sometimes found the wealth of information—and discovering just how much I could do for my child's health—to be overwhelming. Perhaps you feel the same and are wondering where to begin. I think the key is to take it step by step and address the most important issues first, rather than trying to do everything at once.

So which of the things we have covered in this book actually make the biggest difference? If you do want to make changes to your lifestyle, where should you start?

To answer this question, Victor and I once more dug into all of the research laid out in this book. We made a list of all the environmental, medical, and lifestyle factors which were covered by the studies, then we grouped and ranked them all by how much they influence the risk of atopic diseases and allergies.[z] You can find the results in the appendix, under "Appendix 3: What Has the Biggest Effect on Asthma, Eczema, and Allergy Risk?" What do the results tell us?

As they say in the Hippocratic Oath, "First, do no harm." If you're starting anywhere, first you'll want to avoid the risk factors that will dramatically raise your child's risk of atopic diseases above the baseline of the general population.

Of these, the largest increase of atopic disease risk is driven by the use of antibiotics. You can protect your microbiome, and thus your child's, by only taking antibiotics when they are deemed absolutely necessary by your doctor or healthcare provider. Antibiotics can be lifesavers, but using them during

---

[z] Statisticians and epidemiologists might quibble that this is an apples and oranges comparison. Indeed, it is. The studies listed in the table differ with respect to their subject areas, methodology, and sample sizes. But that doesn't mean that it's impossible to compare apples and oranges. If you are not convinced, I refer you to the breakthrough paper "Comparing Apples and Oranges: A randomised Prospective Study" published in the *British Medical Journal*.[666]

pregnancy and in early life can *triple or nearly quadruple your child's risk* of asthma. It also increases the risk of eczema and other allergies by around 50 percent. When your doctor prescribes you antibiotics, check to make sure that it is not just a precautionary prescription. If there is any doubt whether you have a viral or bacterial infection, try to get a test that can differentiate between the two. If you *do* have a bacterial infection, discuss with your doctor whether you can wait to see if the symptoms clear up on their own, or whether there are alternative treatment options, as described in chapter 3.

The second-biggest driver of atopy and allergy risk increases are household/cleaning chemicals and pesticides. Try to minimise your exposure to these types of chemicals, as high exposure can *double or triple your child's risk* of asthma, allergies, and birth defects. Swap your cleaning products and cosmetics, especially sprays, aerosols, and scented products, for more natural alternatives. If you live in a rural area near farms that spray pesticides or herbicides, try to avoid those chemicals as best you can. You can find more details in chapter 9.

Avoiding these major risk factors—antibiotics, toxic household/cleaning chemicals, and pesticides—is a very good start. Next, let's look at the most powerful tools to bring your child's atopy and allergy risk *below* the baseline to near zero.

The strongest protective effects come from taking high-quality supplements (but remember to check with your healthcare provider before you do). The supplements with the biggest positive impact are probiotics and prebiotic fibre, fish oil, folic acid, and vitamin D. Taking these could *prevent up to nine out of ten cases* of eczema and allergies. See chapter 7 for more details.

Yet, supplements come with downsides. For one, high-quality supplements are very expensive (but then, so is having kids!). Low-quality supplements are, at best, a waste of your money; at worst, they could do more harm than good if they contain impurities, preservatives, sweeteners, or other bad stuff. Supplements might also tempt you to think that they're a replacement for eating healthily. They're most definitely not—that's why they're called "supplements" and not "replacements." If I had to pick between eating a healthy diet and taking supplements for maximum health benefits, I'd choose a healthy diet—which is nearly tied with supplements in their ability to prevent chronic disease.

In particular, focus on healthy fats and fibre: fish, olive oil, avocados, nuts, legumes, and whole grains. Time to dust off your Mediterranean cuisine cookbooks! Likewise, consume fermented foods with live bacteria—like yoghurt, sauerkraut, kimchi, kombucha, and kefir. Make sure to introduce fermented foods, especially yoghurt, to your child's diet as early as possible during their first year of life. These steps lower your child's risk of asthma, eczema, and allergies *by up to 85 percent*, meaning that *eight to nine out of ten cases could be prevented*. The details are in chapters 4–6. Granted, out of everything in this book, "eating a healthy diet" is the one that requires the most effort to implement, but it also carries the most long-term benefit. If nothing else, start with baby steps, and "do no harm." Cut out junk food, bad fats, and sugar as much as you can, and gradually make healthier choices. It's easy to feel deflated and think "Oh well, it doesn't matter now" if you've had a couple of bad days, but keep trying. Each meal is a new opportunity to choose something that's better for you and your child, and over time, it'll become second nature.

The next major opportunity to lower your child's risk of chronic illness comes after they are born. Exclusive breastfeeding for four to six months and continued breastfeeding during and after introducing solids for as long as you can could *prevent up to six out of ten cases* of asthma, eczema, and allergies. As we saw in chapter 11, breastfeeding boosts your child's overall health, physical and intellectual development, and budding immune system. It also lets you share your immune defences with your baby. As a result, breastfeeding could *prevent five out of ten cases* of early childhood death, *four out of ten cases* of common childhood cancers, and *five out of ten cases* of Crohn's disease, ulcerative colitis, and celiac disease. It strengthens your bond with your baby, potentially enhances your baby's intelligence for life, gives you more sleep, and it saves you money. If breastfeeding isn't an option for whatever reason, you can still lower your baby's allergy risk by choosing partially or fully hydrolysed formula with added prebiotics instead of regular cow's milk formula, and by avoiding soy formula. This too could *prevent around four out of ten* cases of asthma, eczema, and allergies.

More generally, the studies in this book highlight the benefits of increasing your microbial diversity and that of your baby. Spend time in nature and get dirty. Don't obsess over cleanliness. Visit farms with livestock, preferably organic ones, and—seriously—pet some cows and play with dogs! Besides reducing your stress levels, exposure to farm animals and pets could *prevent up to four out of ten cases* of asthma, eczema, and allergies. To further increase your baby's chances of good health, try to give birth vaginally, and delay the cord clamping by a few minutes. Should you have to give birth by C-section for medical reasons, consider the seeding method to transfer your vaginal microbiome to your baby.

If I had to boil it down to a single sentence, I'd say: avoid harmful chemicals, mind your microbiome, and eat well.

The devil may be in the details, but in the grand scheme of things, it isn't any more complicated than that.

Meanwhile, research continues to progress. We keep improving our understanding of chronic illness and how to free ourselves from its burden. There is a steady stream of new insights into how we, and our children, can live healthier, happier lives. It's my mission to keep learning and sharing what I learn. To stay up to date with the latest discoveries, join me and our community of parents at **www.growhealthybabies.com**!

Last but not least, thank you for reading. I am deeply grateful that you shared your time with me. This is my first book, and I hope you have found it useful. If you did, I would truly appreciate it if you could leave a review of the book wherever you bought it. This would make a huge difference in helping other parents discover it and hopefully benefit from it as well.

I do hope you stay in touch, and I wish you success, good luck, and most of all, joy on your journey through parenthood!

ACKNOWLEDGEMENTS

We are grateful to Simone Davies for her friendship, encouragement, writing and publishing advice, and in-depth notes on our first draft. Her wonderful book *The Montessori Toddler* has been an enormous inspiration to us. A big thank you to Heather Davis for her invaluable reader comments, daily chats, and thoughtful questions; she has made this a much better book. Likewise, we are indebted to Richard Burton and Daria Timoshicheva Fennelly for reading our manuscript and providing insightful feedback and many improvements. Our thanks also go to Zach Obront and our editors Nicole Jobe and Hal Clifford at Scribe Media for shepherding this book into existence.

To our friends scattered near and far who have listened to us talk about this book for the last five years—we've made it; it's finally here! Thank you for sharing in our frustrations and excitement as we laboured and offering us your encouragement and your advice. Arianne, Sanna, David, Arne and Julia, Alex, Jan, Daniela and Dennis—we love you all. And thank you, Mike, for introducing us to each other in the first place!

Just as we were starting to lose hope about Michelle being able to breastfeed our child, Myrte van Lonkhuijsen cycled into our lives. Her kindness and skill helped Michelle and our daughter to start their long and happy breastfeeding journey, for which we are forever grateful, and she remains a dear friend.

A special place in our hearts belongs to Norway and the people who have helped us make this our adopted home. Johanna and Jonathan, Sindre and Marte, and Lowan—thank you for offering us the warmest friendship, thought-provoking chats, and welcoming us to live in a fantastic community that inspires us every day. Aslak and Aina, Hanne and Joakim—you have been the best next-door neighbours we could have asked for.

A special thank you to our parents, Doreen, Hugh, Harry, and Im-Sook, and our extended family in Ireland and Germany for your love and support. We couldn't have achieved any of this without you.

To our daughter—you're the heart and soul of everything we do. We're honoured to be your parents and to share your life. You're the inspiration for us to write this book and so much more. We love you, all the way to Pluto and back!

APPENDIX I

UNDERSTANDING THE CONCEPT OF RELATIVE RISK AND ABSOLUTE RISK

If you're anything like me, words like "statistics," "probability," and "risk" might trigger heart palpitations and bad memories of high school maths tests. No sweat—all you need in order to understand the concept of "relative risk" is basic fifth-grade arithmetic like fractions and divisions. Let's walk through an example so you can see for yourself!

Say we are interested in finding out whether taking antibiotics during pregnancy raises the child's risk of developing asthma later in life. This is the question a cohort study in Copenhagen, Denmark, sought to answer by following the health outcomes of 411 babies for a period of five years after birth.[107] Their mothers all had a history of asthma.

Sixty-three of the 411 babies were exposed to antibiotics during the third trimester of pregnancy—let's call this the "antibiotics group." The remaining 348 babies were not exposed to antibiotics in the womb—let's call this the "no-antibiotics group." The results after five years:

- Of the babies in the antibiotics group, about **one in four** experienced at least one asthma attack by the age of five, which means their probability of developing asthma was **25 percent.**
- Of the babies in the no-antibiotics group, however, only about **one in eight** experienced an asthma attack by the age of five, which means a probability of **12.5 percent.**[aa]

Here's a visual summary:

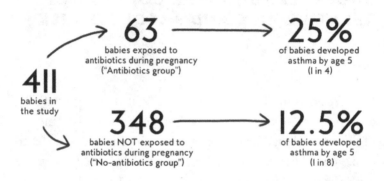

Now, these percentages—25 percent asthma in the antibiotics group and 12.5 percent asthma in the no-antibiotics group—describe what's called absolute risk: a child's overall risk of developing asthma, depending on whether or not they were exposed to antibiotics in the womb. What if you want to compare the asthma risk *between* the two groups? Clearly, the risk in the antibiotics group is much higher, twice as high in this case. Researchers call this relative risk.

---

aa If your memory of fractions, percentages, and probability is a bit rusty, here's a little refresher. Probabilities like "one in four" can be written as a fraction: ¼. You can turn fractions into percentages by dividing the top part by the bottom part, then multiplying by 100: 1 divided by 4 is 0.25, multiplied by 100 equals 25. Thus, ¼ equals 25 percent. So if one in four babies develop asthma, that means 25 percent, or 25 out of 100 babies ("percent" literally means "per hundred") do. One more example: if the probability is one in eight, that means ⅛ = 12.5 percent. When the probability of developing asthma is 12.5 percent, that means about twelve to thirteen out of one hundred kids will develop asthma.

Relative risk is simply calculated by dividing the absolute risk of one group by the absolute risk of the other group. In this example, the relative risk is 25 percent divided by 12.5 percent = 2. This means that children exposed to antibiotics during the third trimester are two times as likely to develop asthma before the age of five. Another way of putting it is that exposure to antibiotics *doubled* the children's risk of developing asthma. Here's the summary of how you get from absolute risk to relative risk:

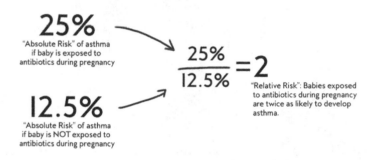

25%
"Absolute Risk" of asthma
if baby is exposed to
antibiotics during pregnancy

12.5%
"Absolute Risk" of asthma
if baby is NOT exposed to
antibiotics during pregnancy

$$\frac{25\%}{12.5\%} = 2$$

"Relative Risk": Babies exposed
to antibiotics during pregnancy
are twice as likely to develop
asthma.

Let's assume that the risk of asthma had been the same in both groups, e.g., 25 percent. Then the relative risk would be 25 percent divided by 25 percent = 1. A relative risk of 1 would mean that there is *no difference* between the groups and that taking antibiotics during pregnancy has no effect on the baby's asthma risk.

And what if the risk of asthma had actually been lower in the antibiotics group? Imagine a result where 12.5 percent of children in the antibiotics group had developed asthma versus 25 percent in the no-antibiotics group. Then the relative risk would be 12.5 percent divided by 25 percent = 0.5. We would say that exposure to antibiotics during pregnancy reduces the child's risk of developing asthma by 50 percent, or by half.

What if the relative risk isn't a neat round number where we can say that the risk "halved" or "doubled," e.g., what if the relative risk is 1.25? Then we would say that the risk is 1.25 times higher, or 25 percent higher, because if you multiply a number by 1.25, you increase it by 25 percent. If the relative risk is 0.75, we would say the risk is 25 percent lower, because if you multiply a number by 0.75, you decrease it by 25 percent.

APPENDIX 2

NUTRIENTS COMMONLY DEFICIENT DURING PREGNANCY AND THEIR EFFECTS ON ASTHMA, ECZEMA, AND ALLERGY RISK

NUTRIENT AND RECOMMENDED DAILY ALLOWANCE (RDA) DURING PREGNANCY AND BREASTFEEDING	OUTCOME
FOLATE (VITAMIN B9) 400-800 µg/day, ideally as L-methylfolate	Lowers the risk of **birth defects** by 70-90 percent[364,365]
VITAMIN D 600 IU/day, but researchers recommend to increase the RDA to 7,000 IU/day	Lowers the risk of **gestational diabetes** by 50 percent and of **preeclampsia** by 70 percent[375] May reduce the risk of **asthma** and **eczema**[361,380,381]
IRON 27 mg/day but ideally more	Lowers the risk of **asthma** and **allergies** by 30-35 percent[388] Improves **brain development** and **IQ**[390,391]

NUTRIENT AND RECOMMENDED DAILY ALLOWANCE (RDA) DURING PREGNANCY AND BREASTFEEDING	OUTCOME
ZINC II mg/day during pregnancy and I2 mg/day during breastfeeding but ideally more	Lowers the risk of **asthma** by 50 percent and of **eczema** by 33 percent when RDA is exceeded[397,398]
IODINE 250 µg/day during pregnancy and 290 µg/day during breastfeeding	Lowers the risk of **physical and mental retardation**[402,403]
CHOLINE 450 mg/day during pregnancy and 550 mg/day during breastfeeding	Lowers the risk of **birth defects** and **learning/memory problems**[409,410]
VITAMIN E I5 mg/day during pregnancy and I9 mg/day during breastfeeding	Lowers the risk of **asthma** by 50 percent[361,397]
PROBIOTICS I0 billion viable organisms (CFU)/day, a mix containing *L. rhamnosus* or *L. paracasei* and *B. longum, B. lactis,* or *B. breve*; also unsweetened yoghurt with live cultures or other fermented foods	Lowers the risk of **eczema** by 50-70 percent[417,418] Lowers the risk of **allergies** by I2-40 percent[419,420] Regularly feeding children yoghurt in the first year of life lowers their risk of **eczema** by 30-70 percent and **allergies** by 40-85 percent[186-188] May lower the risk of **asthma** by 20-30 percent[427] Can cure existing **food allergies**[421-423] and improve **asthma symptoms**[424-426]
OMEGA-3 FATTY ACIDS/ DHA (FISH OIL) At least 200-250 mg/day, ideally 400-I,000 mg/per day	Reduces the risk of **eczema** by 40 percent, **allergies** by 34 percent, and **food allergies** by 90 percent[234] Starting to feed children oily fish before the age of one reduces the risk of **asthma** by 25 percent, **allergies** by 25 percent, and **eczema** by 76 percent[235,236] Improves **brain development** and **IQ**[240,241]

You can also find a list of recommended supplements at www.growhealthybabies.com/supplements.

APPENDIX 3

WHAT HAS THE BIGGEST EFFECT ON ASTHMA, ECZEMA, AND ALLERGY RISK?

STUDY	OUTCOME[AB]
TAKING ANTIBIOTICS	
Wjst, M. et al. Early antibiotic treatment and later asthma. Eur. J. Med. Res. 6, 263-271 (2001).	**68-266 percent higher** risk of **asthma** if the child is given one or more courses of **antibiotics** early in life; **199-288 percent higher** risk of **asthma** if the child is given **antibiotics** in the first months to two years of life
Stensballe, L. G., Simonsen, J., Jensen, S. M., Bønnelykke, K. & Bisgaard, H. Use of antibiotics during pregnancy increases the risk of asthma in early childhood. The Journal of Pediatrics 162, 832-838.e3 (2013).	**98 percent higher** risk of **asthma** if the mother takes **antibiotics** in third trimester of pregnancy

---

ab To make the studies more comparable, we converted studies reporting odds ratio (OR) to relative risk (RR) using their data of "non-exposed prevalence" and the Clincalc conversion tool (you can find it via **www.growhealthybabies.com/clincalc**). When a study didn't report "baseline" or "non-exposed prevalence," we estimated it using Centers for Disease Control and Prevention or other prevalence data.

STUDY	OUTCOME[AB]
McKeever, T. M., Lewis, S. A., Smith, C. & Hubbard, R. The importance of prenatal exposures on the development of allergic disease: a birth cohort study using the West Midlands General Practice Database. American Journal of Respiratory and Critical Care Medicine 166, 827-832 (2002).	**17-68 percent higher** risk of **eczema, hay fever/dust allergy, asthma** if the mother takes more than two courses of **antibiotics** during pregnancy
Foliaki, S. et al. Antibiotic use in infancy and symptoms of asthma, rhinoconjunctivitis, and eczema in children 6 and 7 years old: International Study of Asthma and Allergies in Childhood Phase III. Journal of Allergy and Clinical Immunology 124, 982-989 (2009).	**40-49 percent higher** risk of **eczema, asthma, and hay fever/ dust allergy** if the child is given **antibiotics** in the first year of life

EXPOSURE TO HOUSEHOLD CHEMICALS AND PESTICIDES

Herdt-Losavio, M. L. et al. Maternal occupation and the risk of birth defects: an overview from the National Birth Defects Prevention Study. Occup. Environ. Med. 67, 58-66 (2010).	**43-593 percent higher** risk of **birth defects** if the mother works as a full-time janitor/cleaner due to exposure to **cleaning chemicals**
Salam, M. T., Li, Y.-F., Langholz, B., Gilliland, F. D. & Children's Health Study. Early-life environmental risk factors for asthma: findings from the Children's Health Study. Environ. Health Perspect. 112, 760-765 (2004).	**98-198 percent higher** risk of **asthma** if the child is exposed to **pesticides or herbicides** in the first year of life
Zock, J.-P. et al. The use of household cleaning sprays and adult asthma: an international longitudinal study. Am. J. Respir. Crit. Care Med. 176, 735-741 (2007).	**49-196 percent higher** risk of developing adult **asthma** if using **spray cleaners** at least once a week or three different types of sprays at least once a week for nine years
Savage, J. H., Matsui, E. C., Wood, R. A. & Keet, C. A. Urinary levels of triclosan and parabens are associated with aeroallergen and food sensitization. J. Allergy Clin. Immunol. 130, 453-60.e7 (2012).	**63-172 percent higher** risk of **allergies** if the child has a high exposure to **triclosan or parabens**

STUDY	OUTCOME[AB]
Sherriff, A., Farrow, A., Golding, J. & Henderson, J. Frequent use of chemical household products is associated with persistent wheezing in pre-school age children. Thorax 60, 45-49 (2005).	**120 percent higher** risk of **asthma** if the mother uses high amount of **cleaning products** during pregnancy
Bertelsen, R. J. et al. Triclosan exposure and allergic sensitization in Norwegian children. Allergy 68, 84-91 (2013).	**52-60 percent higher** risk of **allergies and hay fever/dust allergy** if the child has a high exposure to **triclosan**

PROBIOTICS/PREBIOTICS, FISH OIL, VITAMIN AND MINERAL SUPPLEMENTS, AND COMMON NUTRIENT DEFICIENCIES

Chawes, B. L. et al. Cord blood 25(OH)-vitamin D deficiency and childhood asthma, allergy and eczema: the COPSAC2000 birth cohort study. PLoS One 9, e99856 (2014).	**165 percent higher** risk of **lung problems** if the child is **vitamin D deficient** at birth, as measured in cord blood
Gunaratne, A. W., Makrides, M. & Collins, C. T. Maternal prenatal and/or postnatal n-3 long chain polyunsaturated fatty acids (LCPUFA) supplementation for preventing allergies in early childhood. Cochrane Database Syst. Rev. 7, CD010085 (2015).	**39-87 percent lower** risk of **eczema, allergies, and food allergies** if the mother takes **Omega-3 (fish oil) supplements** during pregnancy
Arslanoglu, S. et al. Early dietary intervention with a mixture of prebiotic oligosaccharides reduces the incidence of allergic manifestations and infections during the first two years of life. J. Nutr. 138, 1091-1095 (2008).	**51-85 percent lower** risk of **eczema, asthma, or allergic hives** if the child is given formula with **prebiotic fibre** instead of regular formula
Tang, M. L. K. et al. Administration of a probiotic with peanut oral immunotherapy: A randomized trial. J. Allergy Clin. Immunol. 135, 737-44.e8 (2015).	**81 percent lower** risk of **peanut allergy** if child is given increasing doses of peanut protein with **probiotic supplements**

STUDY	OUTCOME[AB]
Ivakhnenko, O. S. & Nyankovskyy, S. L. Effect of the specific infant formula mixture of oligosaccharides on local immunity and development of allergic and infectious disease in young children: randomized study. Pediatr. Pol. 88, 398-404 (2013).	**63 percent lower** risk of allergic **asthma, 71 percent lower** risk of **eczema**, and 71-76 percent lower risk of food **allergies** if the child is given formula with **prebiotic fibre** instead of standard formula
Berni Canani, R. et al. Effect of Lactobacillus GG on tolerance acquisition in infants with cow's milk allergy: a randomized trial. J. Allergy Clin. Immunol. 129, 580-2, 582.e1-5 (2012).	**78 percent lower** risk of **cow's milk allergy** if the child is given **probiotic supplements** in hypoallergenic formula
Aghajafari, F. et al. Association between maternal serum 25-hydroxyvitamin D level and pregnancy and neonatal outcomes: systematic review and meta-analysis of observational studies. BMJ 346, f1169 (2013).	**45 percent higher** risk of **gestational diabetes** and **72 percent higher** risk of **preeclampsia** if the mother is **vitamin D** deficient
Enomoto, T. et al. Effects of Bifidobacterial supplementation to pregnant women and infants in the prevention of allergy development in infants and on fecal microbiota. Allergol. Int. (2014). doi: 10.2332/allergolint.13-OA-0683	**64-69 percent lower** risk of **eczema** if the mother takes **probiotic supplements** during pregnancy *and* gives them to child after birth
Wickens, K. et al. A protective effect of Lactobacillus rhamnosus HN001 against eczema in the first 2 years of life persists to age 4 years. Clin. Exp. Allergy 42, 1071-1079 (2012).	**43-62 percent lower** risk of **eczema** and **hay fever/dust allergy** if the mother takes **probiotic supplements** during pregnancy *and* gives them to child after birth
Rautava, S., Salminen, S. & Isolauri, E. Specific probiotics in reducing the risk of acute infections in infancy–a randomised, double-blind, placebo-controlled study. Br. J. Nutr. 101, 1722-1726 (2009).	**49-56 percent lower** risk of **ear and respiratory infections** if the child is given **probiotic supplements** daily

STUDY	OUTCOME[AB]
Mansfield, J. A., Bergin, S. W., Cooper, J. R. & Olsen, C. H. Comparative probiotic strain efficacy in the prevention of eczema in infants and children: a systematic review and meta-analysis. Mil. Med. 179, 580–592 (2014).	**26–52 percent lower** risk of **eczema** if the child is given **probiotic supplements** early in life
Devereux, G. et al. Low maternal vitamin E intake during pregnancy is associated with asthma in 5-year-old children. Am. J. Respir. Crit. Care Med. 174, 499–507 (2006).	**33–49 percent lower** risk of **asthma and eczema** if the mother has a high intake of **vitamin E and zinc** during pregnancy
Litonjua, A. A. et al. Maternal antioxidant intake in pregnancy and wheezing illnesses in children at 2 y of age. Am. J. Clin. Nutr. 84, 903–911 (2006).	**47 percent lower** risk of **asthma** if the mother has a high intake of **vitamin E and zinc** during pregnancy
Panduru, M., Panduru, N. M., Salavastru, C. M. & Tiplica, G.-S. Probiotics and primary prevention of atopic dermatitis: a meta-analysis of randomized controlled studies. J. Eur. Acad. Dermatol. Venereol. (2014). doi: 10.1111/jdv.12496	**40–42 percent lower** risk of **eczema** if the mother takes **probiotic supplements** during pregnancy *and* gives them to child after birth
Kuitunen, M. et al. Probiotics prevent IgE-associated allergy until age 5 years in cesarean-delivered children but not in the total cohort. J. Allergy Clin. Immunol. 123, 335–341 (2009).	**40 percent lower** risk of **allergies** if the child born by C-section is given **probiotic supplements**
Miyake, Y., Sasaki, S., Tanaka, K. & Hirota, Y. Dairy food, calcium and vitamin D intake in pregnancy, and wheeze and eczema in infants. Eur. Respir. J. 35, 1228–1234 (2010).	**34–35 percent lower** risk of **eczema and asthma** symptoms if the mother has a high intake of **vitamin D** intake during pregnancy
Nwaru, B. I. et al. An exploratory study of the associations between maternal iron status in pregnancy and childhood wheeze and atopy. Br. J. Nutr. 112, 2018–2027 (2014).	**28–35 percent higher** risk of **allergies and asthma** symptoms if the mother is **iron deficient** at birth or in the first trimester

STUDY	OUTCOME[AB]
Elazab, N. et al. Probiotic administration in early life, atopy, and asthma: a meta-analysis of clinical trials. Pediatrics 132, e666-76 (2013).	**12-14 percent lower** risk of **allergies** if the mother takes **probiotic supplements** during pregnancy or gives them to child after birth

DIET CHOICES

Sausenthaler, S. et al. Margarine and butter consumption, eczema and allergic sensitization in children. The LISA birth cohort study. Pediatr. Allergy Immunol. 17, 85-93 (2006).	**90-100 percent higher** risk of **eczema and allergies** if the child eats **margarine** instead of butter
Fitzsimon, N. et al. Mothers' dietary patterns during pregnancy and risk of asthma symptoms in children at 3 years. Ir. Med. J. 100, suppl 27-32 (2007).	**66-88 percent higher** risk of **asthma** if the mother eats high amounts of **margarine** and similar spreadable fats during pregnancy
Crane, J. et al. Is yoghurt an acceptable alternative to raw milk for reducing eczema and allergy in infancy? Clin. Exp. Allergy 48, 604-606 (2018).	**70-85 percent lower** risk of **eczema** and **allergies** if the child eats **yoghurt** more than once a week between six to twelve months of age
Thorburn, A. N. et al. Evidence that asthma is a developmental origin disease influenced by maternal diet and bacterial metabolites. Nat. Commun. 6, 7320 (2015).	**57-78 percent lower** risk of **asthma** symptoms if the mother has above-average acetate levels due to high **dietary fibre** intake
Oien, T., Storrø, O. & Johnsen, R. Do early intake of fish and fish oil protect against eczema and doctor-diagnosed asthma at 2 years of age? A cohort study. J. Epidemiol. Community Health 64, 124-129 (2010).	**76 percent lower** risk of **eczema** if the child eats **oily fish** at least once a week, starting in the first year of life
Nurmatov, U., Devereux, G. & Sheikh, A. Nutrients and foods for the primary prevention of asthma and allergy: systematic review and meta-analysis. J. Allergy Clin. Immunol. 127, 724-33.e1-30 (2011).	**29-40 percent lower** risk of **allergy and asthma** symptoms if the mother has a high intake of **vitamin D or E** during pregnancy; **41-75 percent lower** risk of **allergy and asthma** symptoms if the mother follows a **Mediterranean diet** during pregnancy

STUDY	OUTCOME[AB]
Chatzi, L. et al. Mediterranean diet in pregnancy is protective for wheeze and atopy in childhood. Thorax 63, 507-513 (2008).	**40-75 percent lower** risk of **allergies and asthma** if the mother follows a **Mediterranean diet** during pregnancy
Bédard, A., Northstone, K., Henderson, A. J. & Shaheen, S. O. Maternal intake of sugar during pregnancy and childhood respiratory and atopic outcomes. Eur. Respir. J. 50, (2017).	**31-75 percent higher risk** of **asthma and allergies** if the mother eats high amount of **sugar** during pregnancy
Roduit, C. et al. Development of atopic dermatitis according to age of onset and association with early-life exposures. J. Allergy Clin. Immunol. 130, 130-6.e5 (2012).	**55 percent lower** risk of **eczema** if the child ate **yoghurt** in the first year of life
Shoda, T. et al. Yogurt consumption in infancy is inversely associated with atopic dermatitis and food sensitization at 5 years of age: a hospital-based birth cohort study. J. Dermatol. Sci. 86, 90-96 (2017).	**27-43 percent lower** risk of **eczema** and **food allergies** at five years of age if the child regularly eats **yoghurt** during first year of life
Yang, H., Xun, P. & He, K. Fish and fish oil intake in relation to risk of asthma: a systematic review and meta-analysis. PLoS One 8, e80048 (2013).	**25 percent lower** risk of **asthma** if the child eats high amounts of **fish** in the first year of life

BREASTFEEDING

Saarinen, U. M. & Kajosaari, M. Breastfeeding as prophylaxis against atopic disease: prospective follow-up study until 17 years old. Lancet 346, 1065-1069 (1995).	**109 percent higher** risk of **atopic diseases** at age one, and **55 percent higher** risk of **atopic diseases** at age seventeen, if the child is **breastfed for less than one month** compared to more than six months
Klopp, A. et al. Modes of infant feeding and the risk of childhood asthma: a prospective birth cohort study. J. Pediatr. 190, 192-199.e2 (2017).	**95 percent higher** risk of **asthma** if the child is **formula-fed** instead of breastfed exclusively for the first three months

STUDY	OUTCOME[AB]
Duijts, L., Ramadhani, M. K. & Moll, H. A. Breastfeeding protects against infectious diseases during infancy in industrialized countries. A systematic review. Matern. Child Nutr. 5, 199–210 (2009).	**20–80 percent lower** risk of **infections, diarrhoea, or hospitalisation** for respiratory infections if the child is being **breastfed**
Ehlayel, M. S. & Bener, A. Duration of breast-feeding and the risk of childhood allergic diseases in a developing country. Allergy Asthma Proc. 29, 386–391 (2008).	**42–71 percent higher** risk of **asthma, allergic rhinitis, and eczema** if the child is **formula-fed** instead of breastfed exclusively for the first six months
Duijts, L., Jaddoe, V. W. V., Hofman, A. & Moll, H. A. Prolonged and exclusive breastfeeding reduces the risk of infectious diseases in infancy. Pediatrics 126, e18–25 (2010).	**25–57 percent lower** risk of **respiratory and gastrointestinal infections** if the child is being **breastfed** exclusively for at least four months
Klement, E., Cohen, R. V., Boxman, J., Joseph, A. & Reif, S. Breastfeeding and risk of inflammatory bowel disease: a systematic review with meta-analysis. Am. J. Clin. Nutr. 80, 1342–1352 (2004).	**46–55 percent lower** risk of **Crohn's disease or ulcerative colitis** if the child is being **breastfed**
Hörnell, A., Lagström, H., Lande, B. & Thorsdottir, I. Breastfeeding, introduction of other foods and effects on health: a systematic literature review for the 5th Nordic Nutrition Recommendations. Food Nutr. Res. 57, (2013).	**52 percent lower** risk of **celiac disease** if the child is introduced to gluten while still being **breastfed**
Gdalevich, M., Mimouni, D. & Mimouni, M. Breast-feeding and the risk of bronchial asthma in childhood: a systematic review with meta-analysis of prospective studies. J. Pediatr. 139, 261–266 (2001).	**27–44 percent lower** risk of **asthma** if the child is **breastfed** exclusively for at least three months
Chen, A. & Rogan, W. J. Breastfeeding and the risk of postneonatal death in the United States. Pediatrics 113, e435–9 (2004).	**16–41 percent lower** risk of child **dying** in the first year of life if it is being **breastfed** instead of formula-fed

STUDY	OUTCOME[AB]
Martin, R. M., Gunnell, D., Owen, C. G. & Smith, G. D. Breast-feeding and childhood cancer: a systematic review with meta-analysis. Int. J. Cancer 117, 1020–1031 (2005).	**9-41 percent lower** risk of common **childhood cancers** like leukaemia, Hodgkin's disease, or neuroblastoma if the child is **breastfed**
Hörnell, A., Lagström, H., Lande, B. & Thorsdottir, I. Breastfeeding, introduction of other foods and effects on health: a systematic literature review for the 5th Nordic Nutrition Recommendations. Food Nutr. Res. 57 (2013).	**20-40 percent lower** risk of **diabetes** if the child is **breastfed** instead of formula-fed
Gdalevich, M., Mimouni, D., David, M. & Mimouni, M. Breast-feeding and the onset of atopic dermatitis in childhood: a systematic review and meta-analysis of prospective studies. J. Am. Acad. Dermatol. 45, 520–527 (2001).	**29-38 percent lower** risk of **eczema** if the child is **breastfed** exclusively for at least three months
Kull, I., Wickman, M., Lilja, G., Nordvall, S. L. & Pershagen, G. Breast feeding and allergic diseases in infants–a prospective birth cohort study. Arch. Dis. Child. 87, 478–481 (2002).	**15-29 percent lower** risk of **asthma, eczema, hay fever/dust allergy, or multiple allergies** if the child is **breastfed** exclusively for at least four months
Oddy, W. H. et al. Association between breast feeding and asthma in 6-year-old children: findings of a prospective birth cohort study. BMJ 319, 815–819 (1999).	**21-24 percent higher** risk of **asthma and allergies** at age six if any **formula** was introduced before the age of four months
Woo, J. G. & Martin, L. J. Does breastfeeding protect against childhood obesity? Moving beyond observational evidence. Curr. Obes. Rep. 4, 207–216 (2015).	**10-20 percent lower** risk of **obesity** if the child is **breastfed**
Amitay, E. L. & Keinan-Boker, L. Breastfeeding and childhood leukemia incidence: a meta-analysis and systematic review. JAMA Pediatr. 169, e151025 (2015).	**9-20 percent lower** risk of **childhood leukaemia** if the child is **breastfed**, especially for longer than six months

TYPE OF FORMULA FED TO BABY

STUDY	OUTCOME[a][b]
Strom, B. L. et al. Exposure to soy-based formula in infancy and endocrinological and reproductive outcomes in young adulthood. JAMA 286, 807–814 (2001).	**71 percent higher** risk of **asthma and allergies** if the child is given **soy formula** instead of cow's milk formula
Szajewska, H. & Horvath, A. A partially hydrolyzed 100 percent whey formula and the risk of eczema and any allergy: an updated meta-analysis. World Allergy Organ. J. 10, 27 (2017).	**9–38 percent lower** risk of **eczema and allergies** if the child is given **partially hydrolysed formula** instead of cow's milk formula

EXPOSURE TO NATURE, ANIMALS, AND DIRT

Campbell, B. E. et al. Exposure to "farming" and objective markers of atopy: a systematic review and meta-analysis. Clin. Exp. Allergy 45, 744–757 (2015).	**36 percent lower** risk of **allergies** if the child is exposed to **farm animals** before age one
Lynch, S. V. et al. Effects of early-life exposure to allergens and bacteria on recurrent wheeze and atopy in urban children. J. Allergy Clin. Immunol. 134, 593–601.e12 (2014).	**30 percent lower** risk of **asthma** symptoms if the child is exposed to **cockroach, mouse, or cat allergens** early in life
Hesselmar, B., Hicke-Roberts, A. & Wennergren, G. Allergy in children in hand versus machine dishwashing. Pediatrics 135, e590-7 (2015).	**21–34 percent lower** risk of **eczema, asthma, hay fever/dust allergy** if child's parents are **hand-washing dishes**, eating/**serving fermented foods**, buying food from a **local farm**

BIRTH BY C-SECTION

Bager, P., Wohlfahrt, J. & Westergaard, T. Caesarean delivery and risk of atopy and allergic disease: meta-analyses. Clin. Exp. Allergy 38, 634–642 (2008).	**15–26 percent higher** risk of **asthma, hay fever/dust allergy, or food allergy** if the child is born by **C-section**
Thavagnanam, S., Fleming, J., Bromley, A., Shields, M. D. & Cardwell, C. R. A meta-analysis of the association between caesarean section and childhood asthma. Clinical & Experimental Allergy 38, 629–633 (2008).	**17 percent higher** risk of **asthma** if the child is born by **C-section**

STUDY	OUTCOME[ab]
O'Neill, S. M. et al. Birth by caesarean section and the risk of adult psychosis: a population-based cohort study. Schizophr. Bull. 42, 633–641 (2016).	**13–17 percent higher** risk of **psychosis, schizophrenia, bipolar disorder, and depression** if the child is born by **C-section**

REFERENCES

1. American College of Allergy Asthma & Immunology. Children with Allergy, Asthma May Be at Higher Risk for ADHD. (2013). Available at: http://acaai.org/news/children-allergy-asthma-may-be-higher-risk-adhd.

2. Zhang, J. & Yu, K. F. What's the relative risk? A method of correcting the odds ratio in cohort studies of common outcomes. *JAMA* 280, 1690–1691 (1998).

3. Kane, S. P. Odds Ratio to Risk Ratio Conversion. (2019). Available at: https://clincalc.com/stats/convertor.aspx. (Accessed: 13th February 2019)

4. WHO. Asthma—Fact Sheet. (2013). Available at: http://www.who.int/mediacentre/factsheets/fs307/en/.

5. Toscano, W. A., Oehlke, K. P. & Kafoury, R. An Environmental Systems Biology Approach to the Study of Asthma. In *Allergy Frontiers: Future Perspectives* (eds. Pawankar, R., Holgate, S. T. & Rosenwasser, L. J.) 10, 239–253 (Springer Science & Business Media, 2009).

6. Asthma and Allergy Foundation of America. Asthma Facts and Figures. (2015). Available at: http://www.aafa.org/page/Asthma-facts.aspx.

7. WHO. *Prevalence of Asthma and Allergies in Children.* (2007).

8. WHO. Bronchial Asthma—Fact Sheet. (2016). Available at: http://www.who.int/mediacentre/factsheets/fs206/en/.

9. CDC. Asthma. *FastStats* (2015). Available at: http://www.cdc.gov/nchs/fastats/asthma.htm.

10. European Respiratory Society. Childhood Asthma. *European Lung White Book* (2019). Available at: https://www.erswhitebook.org/chapters/childhood-asthma/. (Accessed: 15th February 2019)

11. *The Global Asthma Report.* (Global Asthma Network, 2014).

12. Schonmann, Y. et al. Atopic eczema in adulthood and risk of depression and anxiety: A population-based cohort study. *J. Allergy Clin. Immunol. Pract.* (2019). doi: 10.1016/j.jaip.2019.08.030

13. CDC. QuickStats: Percentage of Children Aged ≤17 Years with Eczema or Any Kind of Skin Allergy, by Selected Races/Ethnicities—National Health Interview Survey, United States, 2000–2010. *Morbidity and Mortality Weekly Report* (2011). Available at: http://www.cdc.gov/mmwr/preview/mmwrhtml/mm6044a9.htm.

14. Dermatology Information System. How Common Is Eczema? *University of Heidelberg, University of Erlangen* (2016). Available at: http://eczema.dermis.net/content/e01geninfo/e03common/index_eng.html.

15. Deckers, I. A. G. et al. Investigating international time trends in the incidence and prevalence of atopic eczema 1990–2010: A systematic review of epidemiological studies. *PLoS One* 7, e39803 (2012).

16. Margolis, J. S., Abuabara, K., Bilker, W., Hoffstad, O. & Margolis, D. J. Persistence of mild to moderate atopic dermatitis. *JAMA Dermatol.* 150, 593–600 (2014).

17. Ker, J. & Hartert, T. V. The atopic march: What's the evidence? *Ann. Allergy Asthma Immunol.* 103, 282–289 (2009).

18. Kapoor, R. et al. The prevalence of atopic triad in children with physician-confirmed atopic dermatitis. *J. Am. Acad. Dermatol.* 58, 68–73 (2008).

19. Ratini, M. Allergy Statistics and Facts. *WebMD* (2017). Available at: https://www.webmd.com/allergies/allergy-statistics. (Accessed: 19th February 2019)

20. Allergy Statistics & Facts. *Allergy UK* (2019). Available at: https://www.allergyuk.org/information-and-advice/statistics. (Accessed: 19th February 2019)

21. Turner, P. J. et al. Increase in anaphylaxis-related hospitalizations but no increase in fatalities: An analysis of United Kingdom national anaphylaxis data, 1992-2012. *J. Allergy Clin. Immunol.* 135, 956–63.e1 (2015).

22. Castellazzi, A. et al. Probiotics and food allergy. *Ital. J. Pediatr.* 39, 47 (2013).

23. Prescott, S. & Allen, K. J. Food allergy: Riding the second wave of the allergy epidemic. *Pediatr. Allergy Immunol.* 22, 155–160 (2011).

24. Australasian Society of Clinical Immunology and Allergy. Food Allergy. (2016). Available at: http://www.allergy.org.au/patients/food-allergy/food-allergy.

25. Romagnani, S. Th1/Th2 cells. *Inflamm. Bowel Dis.* 5, 285–294 (1999).

26. Romagnani, S. T-cell subsets (Th1 versus Th2). *Ann. Allergy Asthma Immunol.* 85, 9–18; quiz 18, 21 (2000).

27. Berger, A. Th1 and Th2 responses: What are they? *BMJ* 321, 424 (2000).

28. Reinhard, G., Noll, A., Schlebusch, H., Mallmann, P. & Ruecker, A. V. Shifts in the TH1/TH2 balance during human pregnancy correlate with apoptotic changes. *Biochem. Biophys. Res. Commun.* 245, 933–938 (1998).

29. Sykes, L. et al. Changes in the Th1:Th2 Cytokine bias in pregnancy and the effects of the anti-inflammatory cyclopentenone prostaglandin 15-deoxy-Δ 12, 14 -prostaglandin J 2. *Mediators Inflamm.* 2012, 1–12 (2012).

30. Schlanger, Z. Your Microbiome Extends in a Microbial Cloud around You, Like an Aura. *Newsweek* (2015). Available at: https://www.newsweek.com/microbial-cloud-aka-auras-are-basically-real-375010. (Accessed: 18th June 2019)

31. Abbott, A. Scientists bust myth that our bodies have more bacteria than human cells. *Nature* (2016). doi: 10.1038/nature.2016.19136

32. National Institutes of Health. NIH Human Microbiome Project Defines Normal Bacterial Makeup of the Body. (2012). Available at: http://www.nih.gov/news-events/news-releases/nih-human-microbiome-project-defines-normal-bacterial-makeup-body.

33. Konkel, L. The environment within: Exploring the role of the gut microbiome in health and disease. *Environ. Health Perspect.* 121, A276–81 (2013).

34. Genetic Science Learning Center. *The Microbiome and Disease.* (University of Utah, 2016).

35. Vighi, G., Marcucci, F., Sensi, L., Di Cara, G. & Frati, F. Allergy and the gastrointestinal system. *Clinical & Experimental Immunology* 153, 3–6 (2008).

36. Funkhouser, L. J. & Bordenstein, S. R. Mom knows best: The universality of maternal microbial transmission. *PLoS Biol.* 11, e1001631 (2013).

37. Arrieta, M.-C., Stiemsma, L. T., Amenyogbe, N., Brown, E. M. & Finlay, B. The intestinal microbiome in early life: Health and disease. *Front. Immunol.* 5, (2014).

38. Arrieta, M.-C. et al. Early infancy microbial and metabolic alterations affect risk of childhood asthma. *Sci. Transl. Med.* 7, 307ra152 (2015).

39. Jeurink, P. V. et al. Human milk: A source of more life than we imagine. *Benef. Microbes* 4, 17–30 (2013).

40. Cabrera-Rubio, R. et al. The human milk microbiome changes over lactation and is shaped by maternal weight and mode of delivery. *Am. J. Clin. Nutr.* 96, 544–551 (2012).

41. Bäckhed, F. et al. Dynamics and stabilization of the human gut microbiome during the first year of life. *Cell Host Microbe* 17, 690–703 (2015).

42. Bezkorovainy, A. Probiotics: Determinants of survival and growth in the gut. *Am. J. Clin. Nutr.* 73, 399–405 (2001).

43. Liévin, V. et al. Bifidobacterium strains from resident infant human gastrointestinal microflora exert antimicrobial activity. *Gut* 47, 646–652 (2000).

44. Ghadimi, D. et al. Effects of probiotic bacteria and their genomic DNA on TH1/TH2-cytokine production by peripheral blood mononuclear cells (PBMCs) of healthy and allergic subjects. *Immunobiology* 213, 677–692 (2008).

45. Helander, H. F. & Fändriks, L. Surface area of the digestive tract—revisited. *Scand. J. Gastroenterol.* 49, 681–689 (2014).

46. Delmas, J., Dalmasso, G. & Bonnet, R. *Escherichia coli*: The good, the bad and the ugly. *Clinical Microbiology: Open Access* 4, 1–3 (2015).

47. Hasselbalch, H., Jeppesen, D. L., Engelmann, M. D., Michaelsen, K. F. & Nielsen, M. B. Decreased thymus size in formula-fed infants compared with breastfed infants. *Acta Paediatr.* 85, 1029–1032 (1996).

48. Indrio, F., Ladisa, G., Mautone, A. & Montagna, O. Effect of a fermented formula on thymus size and stool pH in healthy term infants. *Pediatr. Res.* 62, 98–100 (2007).

49. Kim, J.-H. et al. Extracellular vesicle-derived protein from *Bifidobacterium longum* alleviates food allergy through mast cell suppression. *J. Allergy Clin. Immunol.* 137, 507–516. e8 (2016).

50. Wu, G. D. et al. Linking long-term dietary patterns with gut microbial enterotypes. *Science* 334, 105–108 (2011).

51. den Besten, G. et al. The role of short-chain fatty acids in the interplay between diet, gut microbiota, and host energy metabolism. *J. Lipid Res.* 54, 2325–2340 (2013).

52. Donohoe, D. R. et al. The microbiome and butyrate regulate energy metabolism and autophagy in the mammalian colon. *Cell Metab.* 13, 517–526 (2011).

53. Tan, J. et al. *The role of short-chain fatty acids in health and disease.* 121, 91–119 (Elsevier Inc., 2014).

54. Böttcher, M. F., Nordin, E. K., Sandin, A., Midtvedt, T. & Björkstén, B. Microflora-associated characteristics in faeces from allergic and nonallergic infants. *Clinical & Experimental Allergy* 30, 1590–1596 (2000).

55. Smith, P. A. The tantalizing links between gut microbes and the brain. *Nature* 526, 312–314 (2015).

56. Young, E. Gut instincts: The secrets of your second brain. *New Scientist* (2012). Available at: https://www.newscientist.com/article/mg21628951.900-gut-instincts-the-secrets-of-your-second-brain/?full=true.

57. Corcoran, C. D., Thomas, P., Phillips, J. & O'Keane, V. Vagus nerve stimulation in chronic treatment-resistant depression: Preliminary findings of an open-label study. *Br. J. Psychiatry* 189, 282–283 (2006).

58. Wall, R. et al. Bacterial neuroactive compounds produced by psychobiotics. In *Microbial Endocrinology: The Microbiota-Gut-Brain Axis in Health and Disease* 817, 221–239 (2014).

59. Tillisch, K. et al. Consumption of fermented milk product with probiotic modulates brain activity. *Gastroenterology* 144, 1394–1401, 1401.e1–4 (2013).

60. Messaoudi, M. et al. Assessment of psychotropic-like properties of a probiotic formulation (*Lactobacillus helveticus* R0052 and *Bifidobacterium longum* R0175) in rats and human subjects. *British Journal of Nutrition* 105, 755–764 (2011).

61. Benton, D., Williams, C. & Brown, A. Impact of consuming a milk drink containing a probiotic on mood and cognition. *European Journal of Clinical Nutrition* 61, 355–361 (2007).

62. Pinto-Sanchez, M. I. et al. Probiotic *Bifidobacterium longum* NCC3001 reduces depression scores and alters brain activity: A pilot study in patients with irritable bowel syndrome. *Gastroenterology* 153, 448–459.e8 (2017).

63. Yang, B., Wei, J., Ju, P. & Chen, J. Effects of regulating intestinal microbiota on anxiety symptoms: A systematic review. *Gen. Psychiatr.* **32**, e100056 (2019).

64. Schmidt, K. et al. Prebiotic intake reduces the waking cortisol response and alters emotional bias in healthy volunteers. *Psychopharmacology* **232**, 1793–1801 (2015).

65. Kohn, D. When gut bacteria changes brain function. Some researchers believe that the microbiome may p... *The Atlantic* (2015).

66. Broad Institute. Transcription Factor. (2016). Available at: https://www.broadinstitute.org/education/glossary/transcription-factor.

67. National Human Genome Research Institute. Epigenomics. *Genome.gov* (2015). Available at: https://www.genome.gov/27532724.

68. Waterland, R. A. & Jirtle, R. L. Transposable elements: Targets for early nutritional effects on epigenetic gene regulation. *Mol. Cell. Biol.* **23**, 5293–5300 (2003).

69. Genetic Science Learning Center. Nutrition and the Epigenome. *Learn.Genetics* (2016). Available at: http://learn.genetics.utah.edu/content/epigenetics/nutrition/.

70. Hoepner, L. A. et al. Bisphenol A and adiposity in an inner-city birth cohort. *Environ. Health Perspect.* **124**, 1644–1650 (2016).

71. Yang, C. Z., Yaniger, S. I., Jordan, V. C., Klein, D. J. & Bittner, G. D. Most plastic products release estrogenic chemicals: A potential health problem that can be solved. *Environ. Health Perspect.* **119**, 989–996 (2011).

72. Blake, M. The Scary New Evidence on BPA-Free Plastics. *Mother Jones* (2014). Available at: http://www.motherjones.com/environment/2014/03/tritan-certichem-eastman-bpa-free-plastic-safe.

73. Joubert, B. R. et al. DNA Methylation in Newborns and Maternal Smoking in Pregnancy: Genome-wide Consortium Meta-analysis. *Am. J. Hum. Genet.* **98**, 680–696 (2016)

74. Hughes, V. Epigenetics: The sins of the father. *Nature* **507**, 22–24 (2014).

75. Day, J., Savani, S., Krempley, B. D., Nguyen, M. & Kitlinska, J. B. Influence of paternal preconception exposures on their offspring: Through epigenetics to phenotype. *Am. J. Stem Cells* **5**, 11–18 (2016).

76. Zhang, S. et al. Parental alcohol consumption and the risk of congenital heart diseases in offspring: An updated systematic review and meta-analysis. *Eur. J. Prev. Cardiol.* 2047487319874530 (2019).

77. European Society of Cardiology. Fathers-to-be should avoid alcohol six months before conception: Parental alcohol consumption linked to raised risk of congenital heart disease. *Science Daily* (2019).

78. Shenderov, B. A. Gut indigenous microbiota and epigenetics. *Microb. Ecol. Health Dis.* **23**, (2012).

79. Türker, N., Toh, Z. Q., Karagiannis, T. C. & Licciardi, P. V. Anti-inflammatory Effects of Probiotics and Their Metabolites: Possible Role for Epigenetic Effects. In *Molecular Mechanisms and Physiology of Disease* 127–150 (Springer New York, 2014).

80. Paparo, L. et al. The influence of early life nutrition on epigenetic regulatory mechanisms of the immune system. *Nutrients* 6, 4706–4719 (2014).

81. Tedelind, S., Westberg, F., Kjerrulf, M. & Vidal, A. Anti-inflammatory properties of the short-chain fatty acids acetate and propionate: A study with relevance to inflammatory bowel disease. *World J. Gastroenterol.* 13, 2826–2832 (2007).

82. Kumar, H. et al. Gut microbiota as an epigenetic regulator: Pilot study based on whole-genome methylation analysis. *MBio* 5, e02113–14 (2014).

83. Berni Canani, R., Di Costanzo, M. & Leone, L. The epigenetic effects of butyrate: Potential therapeutic implications for clinical practice. *Clin. Epigenetics* 4, 4 (2012).

84. Strachan, D. P. Hay fever, hygiene, and household size. *BMJ* 299, 1259–1260 (1989).

85. Wolfe, N. D., Dunavan, C. P. & Diamond, J. *Origins of Major Human Infectious Diseases.* (National Academies Press (US), 2012).

86. Smith, R. S., Bloomfield, S. F. & Rook, G. A. The hygiene hypothesis and its implications for home hygiene, lifestyle and public health. *International Scientific Forum on Home Hygiene* 1–113 (2012).

87. Laursen, M. F. et al. Having older siblings is associated with gut microbiota development during early childhood. *BMC Microbiol.* 15, 154 (2015).

88. Dahl, M. E., Dabbagh, K., Liggitt, D., Kim, S. & Lewis, D. B. Viral-induced T helper type 1 responses enhance allergic disease by effects on lung dendritic cells. *Nat. Immunol.* 5, 337–343 (2004).

89. Umetsu, D. T. Flu strikes the hygiene hypothesis. *Nat. Med.* 10, 88–90 (2004).

90. Fujimura, K. E. & Lynch, S. V. Microbiota in allergy and asthma and the emerging relationship with the gut microbiome. *Cell Host Microbe* 17, 592–602 (2015).

91. Hanski, I. et al. Environmental biodiversity, human microbiota, and allergy are interrelated. *Proc. Natl. Acad. Sci. U.S.A.* 109, 8334–8339 (2012).

92. Wlasiuk, G. & Vercelli, D. The farm effect, or: when, what and how a farming environment protects from asthma and allergic disease. *Curr. Opin. Allergy Clin. Immunol.* 12, 461–466 (2012).

93. von Mutius, E. & Vercelli, D. Farm living: Effects on childhood asthma and allergy. *Nat. Rev. Immunol.* 10, 861–868 (2010).

94. Campbell, B. E. et al. Exposure to "farming" and objective markers of atopy: A systematic review and meta-analysis. *Clin. Exp. Allergy* 45, 744–757 (2015).

95. Lodge, C. J. et al. Perinatal cat and dog exposure and the risk of asthma and allergy in the urban environment: A systematic review of longitudinal studies. *Clin. Dev. Immunol.* 2012, 176484 (2012).

96. Aichbhaumik, N. et al. Prenatal exposure to household pets influences fetal immunoglobulin E production. *Clin. Exp. Allergy* 38, 1787–1794 (2008).

97. Valkonen, M. et al. Bacterial exposures and associations with atopy and asthma in children. *PLoS One* 10, e0131594 (2015).

98. Lynch, S. V. et al. Effects of early-life exposure to allergens and bacteria on recurrent wheeze and atopy in urban children. *J. Allergy Clin. Immunol.* 134, 593–601.e12 (2014).

99. Hesselmar, B., Hicke-Roberts, A. & Wennergren, G. Allergy in children in hand versus machine dishwashing. *Pediatrics* 135, e590–7 (2015).

100. Francino, M. P. Antibiotics and the human gut microbiome: Dysbioses and accumulation of resistances. *Frontiers in Microbiology* 6, 1543 (2015).

101. Jernberg, C., Löfmark, S., Edlund, C. & Jansson, J. K. Long-term ecological impacts of antibiotic administration on the human intestinal microbiota. *ISME Journal* 1, 56–66 (2007).

102. Zaura, E. et al. Same exposure but two radically different responses to antibiotics: Resilience of the salivary microbiome versus long-term microbial shifts in feces. *MBio* 6, e01693–15 (2015).

103. Blaser, M. Antibiotic overuse: Stop the killing of beneficial bacteria. *Nature* 476, 393–394 (2011).

104. Skerrett, P. Doctors prescribe way too many antibiotics. Experts offer tips on cutting back. *STAT* (2016). Available at: https://www.statnews.com/2016/01/19/overprescribing-antibiotics-advice/. (Accessed: 27th April 2016)

105. Foliaki, S. et al. Antibiotic use in infancy and symptoms of asthma, rhinoconjunctivitis, and eczema in children 6 and 7 years old: International Study of Asthma and Allergies in Childhood Phase III. *Journal of Allergy and Clinical Immunology* 124, 982–989 (2009).

106. McKeever, T. M., Lewis, S. A., Smith, C. & Hubbard, R. The importance of prenatal exposures on the development of allergic disease: A birth cohort study using the West Midlands General Practice Database. *American Journal of Respiratory and Critical Care Medicine* 166, 827–832 (2002).

107. Stensballe, L. G., Simonsen, J., Jensen, S. M., Bønnelykke, K. & Bisgaard, H. Use of antibiotics during pregnancy increases the risk of asthma in early childhood. *The Journal of Pediatrics* 162, 832–838.e3 (2013).

108. Wjst, M. et al. Early antibiotic treatment and later asthma. *Eur. J. Med. Res.* 6, 263–271 (2001).

109. Greene, A. Antibiotic Overuse. *DrGreene.com* (2009). Available at: http://www.drgreene.com/qa-articles/antibiotic-overuse/. (Accessed: 28th April 2016)

110. Fleming-Dutra, K. E. et al. Prevalence of inappropriate antibiotic prescriptions among US ambulatory care visits, 2010–2011. *JAMA* 315, 1864–1873 (2016).

111.   Belluz, J. Why doctors overprescribe antibiotics—even in cases where they're useless. *Vox* (2015). Available at: http://www.vox.com/2015/11/27/9802108/doctors-abuse-overprescribe-antibiotics. (Accessed: 26th April 2016)

112.   Ohlsson, A. & Shah, V. S. Intrapartum antibiotics for known maternal Group B streptococcal colonization. In *Cochrane Database of Systematic Reviews* (John Wiley & Sons, Ltd, 1996).

113.   Levine, E. M., Ghai, V., Barton, J. J. & Strom, C. M. Intrapartum antibiotic prophylaxis increases the incidence of Gram-negative neonatal sepsis. *Infect. Dis. Obstet. Gynecol.* 7, 210–213 (1999).

114.   Donders, G. G. G., Zodzika, J. & Rezeberga, D. Treatment of bacterial vaginosis: What we have and what we miss. *Expert Opin. Pharmacother.* 15, 645–657 (2014).

115.   Allsworth, J. E. & Peipert, J. F. Prevalence of bacterial vaginosis: 2001–2004 National Health and Nutrition Examination Survey data. *Obstet. Gynecol.* 109, 114–120 (2007).

116.   Velasquez-Manoff, M. What's in Your Vagina? A Healthy Microbiome, Hopefully. *Slate Magazine* (2013). Available at: http://www.slate.com/articles/health_and_science/ medical_examiner/2013/01/microbial_balance_in_vagina_miscarriage_infertility_pre_ term_birth_linked.html. (Accessed: 2nd May 2016)

117.   Morse, J. Why Douching Won't Die. *The Atlantic.* Available at: http://www.theatlantic.com/ health/archive/2015/04/why-douching-wont-die/390198/. (Accessed: 3rd May 2016)

118.   Cottrell, B. H. An updated review of evidence to discourage douching. *MCN Am. J. Matern. Child Nurs.* 35, 102–107; quiz 108–9 (2010).

119.   Donders, G. G. G. et al. Effect of lyophilized lactobacilli and 0.03 mg estriol (Gynoflor®) on vaginitis and vaginosis with disrupted vaginal microflora: A multicenter, randomized, single-blind, active-controlled pilot study. *Gynecologic and Obstetric Investigation* 70, 264–272 (2010).

120.   Anukam, K. C. et al. Clinical study comparing probiotic Lactobacillus GR-1 and RC-14 with metronidazole vaginal gel to treat symptomatic bacterial vaginosis. *Microbes Infect.* 8, 2772–2776 (2006).

121.   Mastromarino, P. et al. Effectiveness of *Lactobacillus*-containing vaginal tablets in the treatment of symptomatic bacterial vaginosis. *Clin. Microbiol. Infect.* 15, 67–74 (2009).

122.   Menard, J.-P. Antibacterial treatment of bacterial vaginosis: Current and emerging therapies. *Int. J. Women's Health* 3, 295–305 (2011).

123.   Head, K. A. Natural approaches to prevention and treatment of infections of the lower urinary tract. *Altern. Med. Rev.* 13, 227–244 (2008).

124.   Stapleton, A. E. et al. Randomized, placebo-controlled phase 2 trial of a *Lactobacillus crispatus* probiotic given intravaginally for prevention of recurrent urinary tract infection. *Clin. Infect. Dis.* 52, 1212–1217 (2011).

125.   Olesen, C. et al. Drug use in first pregnancy and lactation: A population-based survey among Danish women. The EUROMAP group. *Eur. J. Clin. Pharmacol.* 55, 139–144 (1999).

126. Gabbe, S. G. *Obstetrics: Normal and Problem Pregnancies.* (Elsevier Health Sciences, 2012).

127. Hu, X. et al. *Clostridium tyrobutyricum* alleviates *Staphylococcus aureus*-induced endometritis in mice by inhibiting endometrial barrier disruption and inflammatory response. *Food Funct.* (2019). doi: 10.1039/c9fo00654k

128. Liu, M., Wu, Q., Wang, M., Fu, Y. & Wang, J. *Lactobacillus rhamnosus* GR-1 limits *Escherichia coli*-induced inflammatory responses via attenuating MyD88-dependent and MyD88-independent pathway activation in bovine endometrial epithelial cells. *Inflammation* 39, 1483–1494 (2016).

129. Otero, M. C., Morelli, L. & Nader-Macías, M. E. Probiotic properties of vaginal lactic acid bacteria to prevent metritis in cattle. *Lett. Appl. Microbiol.* 43, 91–97 (2006).

130. Kawakita, T. & Landy, H. J. Surgical site infections after cesarean delivery: Epidemiology, prevention and treatment. *Matern. Health Neonatol. Perinatol.* 3, 12 (2017).

131. Kasatpibal, N. et al. Effectiveness of probiotic, prebiotic, and synbiotic therapies in reducing postoperative complications: A systematic review and network meta-analysis. *Clin. Infect. Dis.* 64, S153–S160 (2017).

132. Angelopoulou, A. et al. The microbiology and treatment of human mastitis. *Med. Microbiol. Immunol.* 207, 83–94 (2018).

133. Arroyo, R. et al. Treatment of infectious mastitis during lactation: Antibiotics versus oral administration of *Lactobacilli* isolated from breast milk. *Clin. Infect. Dis.* 50, 1551–1558 (2010).

134. Jiménez, E. et al. Oral administration of *Lactobacillus* strains isolated from breast milk as an alternative for the treatment of infectious mastitis during lactation. *Appl. Environ. Microbiol.* 74, 4650–4655 (2008).

135. Fernández, L. et al. Prevention of infectious mastitis by oral administration of *Lactobacillus salivarius* PS2 during late pregnancy. *Clin. Infect. Dis.* 62, 568–573 (2016).

136. Hurtado, J. A. et al. Oral administration to nursing women of *Lactobacillus fermentum* CECT5716 prevents lactational mastitis development: A randomized controlled trial. *Breastfeed. Med.* 12, 202 (2017).

137. Mathew, J. L. Effect of maternal antibiotics on breast feeding infants. *Postgrad. Med. J.* 80, 196–200 (2004).

138. Leyer, G. J., Li, S., Mubasher, M. E., Reifer, C. & Ouwehand, A. C. Probiotic effects on cold and influenza-like symptom incidence and duration in children. *Pediatrics* 124, e172–9 (2009).

139. de Vrese, M. et al. Probiotic bacteria reduced duration and severity but not the incidence of common cold episodes in a double blind, randomized, controlled trial. *Vaccine* 24, 6670–6674 (2006).

140. Rautava, S., Salminen, S. & Isolauri, E. Specific probiotics in reducing the risk of acute infections in infancy—a randomised, double-blind, placebo-controlled study. *Br. J. Nutr.* 101, 1722–1726 (2009).

141. Sazawal, S. et al. Prebiotic and probiotic fortified milk in prevention of morbidities among children: Community-based, randomized, double-blind, controlled trial. *PLoS One* 5, e12164 (2010).

142. Makino, S. et al. Reducing the risk of infection in the elderly by dietary intake of yoghurt fermented with *Lactobacillus delbrueckii* ssp. *bulgaricus* OLL1073R-1. *Br. J. Nutr.* 104, 998–1006 (2010).

143. Sugimura, T. et al. Effects of oral intake of plasmacytoid dendritic cells-stimulative lactic acid bacterial strain on pathogenesis of influenza-like illness and immunological response to influenza virus. *Br. J. Nutr.* 114, 727–733 (2015).

144. Meng, H. et al. Consumption of *Bifidobacterium animalis* subsp. *lactis* BB-12 impacts upper respiratory tract infection and the function of NK and T cells in healthy adults. *Mol. Nutr. Food Res.* 60, 1161–1171 (2016).

145. Ringel-Kulka, T., Kotch, J. B., Jensen, E. T., Savage, E. & Weber, D. J. Randomized, double-blind, placebo-controlled study of synbiotic yogurt effect on the health of children. *J. Pediatr.* 166, 1475–81.e1–3 (2015).

146. Henriques, M. Is it worth taking probiotics after antibiotics? *BBC* (2019).

147. Guo, Q., Goldenberg, J. Z., Humphrey, C., El Dib, R. & Johnston, B. C. Probiotics for the prevention of pediatric antibiotic-associated diarrhea. *Cochrane Database Syst. Rev.* 4, CD004827 (2019).

148. Agamennone, V., Krul, C. A. M., Rijkers, G. & Kort, R. A practical guide for probiotics applied to the case of antibiotic-associated diarrhea in the Netherlands. *BMC Gastroenterol.* 18, 103 (2018).

149. Hempel, S. et al. Probiotics for the prevention and treatment of antibiotic-associated diarrhea: A systematic review and meta-analysis. *JAMA* 307, 1959–1969 (2012).

150. Depestel, D. D. & Aronoff, D. M. Epidemiology of *Clostridium difficile* infection. *J. Pharm. Pract.* 26, 464–475 (2013).

151. Goldenberg, J. Z., Mertz, D. & Johnston, B. C. Probiotics to prevent *Clostridium difficile* infection in patients receiving antibiotics. *JAMA* 320, 499–500 (2018).

152. Pattani, R., Palda, V. A., Hwang, S. W. & Shah, P. S. Probiotics for the prevention of antibiotic-associated diarrhea and *Clostridium difficile* infection among hospitalized patients: Systematic review and meta-analysis. *Open Med.* 7, e56–67 (2013).

153. Goldenberg, J. Z. et al. Probiotics for the prevention of *Clostridium difficile*-associated diarrhea in adults and children. *Cochrane Database Syst. Rev.* 12, CD006095 (2017).

154. Issa, I. & Moucari, R. Probiotics for antibiotic-associated diarrhea: Do we have a verdict? *World J. Gastroenterol.* 20, 17788–17795 (2014).

155. Di Cerbo, A., Palmieri, B., Aponte, M., Morales-Medina, J. C. & Iannitti, T. Mechanisms and therapeutic effectiveness of lactobacilli. *J. Clin. Pathol.* 69, 187–203 (2016).

156. Cohen, L. Those Probiotics May Actually Be Hurting Your "Gut Health." *WSJ Online* (2019).

157. Consumer Reports. Are probiotic supplements for your gut really good for you? *The Washington Post* (2019).

158. Suez, J. et al. Post-antibiotic gut mucosal microbiome reconstitution is impaired by probiotics and improved by autologous FMT. *Cell* 174, 1406–1423.e16 (2018).

159. Kabbani, T. A. et al. Prospective randomized controlled study on the effects of *Saccharomyces boulardii* CNCM I-745 and amoxicillin-clavulanate or the combination on the gut microbiota of healthy volunteers. *Gut Microbes* 8, 17–32 (2017).

160. Engelbrektson, A. et al. Probiotics to minimize the disruption of faecal microbiota in healthy subjects undergoing antibiotic therapy. *J. Med. Microbiol.* 58, 663–670 (2009).

161. Hummelen, R. et al. *Lactobacillus rhamnosus* GR-1 and *L. reuteri* RC-14 to prevent or cure bacterial vaginosis among women with HIV. *Int. J. Gynaecol. Obstet.* 111, 245–248 (2010).

162. Rehman, A. et al. Effects of probiotics and antibiotics on the intestinal homeostasis in a computer controlled model of the large intestine. *BMC Microbiol.* 12, 47 (2012).

163. Berstad, A., Raa, J., Midtvedt, T. & Valeur, J. Probiotic lactic acid bacteria—the fledgling cuckoos of the gut? *Microb. Ecol. Health Dis.* 27, 31557 (2016).

164. Spilde, I. Are probiotics really that good for you? *Science Norway* (2016). Available at: https://sciencenorway.no/forskningno-gut-bacteria-norway/are-probiotics-really-that-good-for-you/1434985. (Accessed: 28th October 2019)

165. Lerner, A., Shoenfeld, Y. & Matthias, T. Probiotics: If it does not help it does not do any harm. Really? *Microorganisms* 7 (2019).

166. Suez, J., Zmora, N., Segal, E. & Elinav, E. The pros, cons, and many unknowns of probiotics. *Nat. Med.* 25, 716–729 (2019).

167. Zmora, N. et al. Personalized gut mucosal colonization resistance to empiric probiotics is associated with unique host and microbiome features. *Cell* 174, 1388–1405.e21 (2018).

168. Laursen, M. F. et al. Administration of two probiotic strains during early childhood does not affect the endogenous gut microbiota composition despite probiotic proliferation. *BMC Microbiol.* 17, 175 (2017).

169. David, L. A. et al. Diet rapidly and reproducibly alters the human gut microbiome. *Nature* 505, 559–563 (2014).

170. Gibson, G. R. & Roberfroid, M. B. Dietary modulation of the human colonic microbiota: Introducing the concept of prebiotics. *J. Nutr.* 125, 1401–1412 (1995).

171. Kaczmarczyk, M. M., Miller, M. J. & Freund, G. G. The health benefits of dietary fiber: Beyond the usual suspects of type 2 diabetes mellitus, cardiovascular disease and colon cancer. *Metabolism* 61, 1058–1066 (2012).

172. Harvard School of Public Health. Fiber. *Harvard Nutrition Source* (2012). Available at: http://www.hsph.harvard.edu/nutritionsource/carbohydrates/fiber/. (Accessed: 31st May 2016)

173. Oaklander, M. How Changing Your Diet Changes Your Gut Bacteria. *Time* (2015).

174. Clemens, R. et al. Filling America's fiber intake gap: Summary of a roundtable to probe realistic solutions with a focus on grain-based foods. *J. Nutr.* 142, 1390S–401S (2012).

175. Fedirko, V. et al. Glycemic index, glycemic load, dietary carbohydrate, and dietary fiber intake and risk of liver and biliary tract cancers in Western Europeans. *Ann. Oncol.* 24, 543–553 (2013).

176. Eaton, S. B. The ancestral human diet: What was it and should it be a paradigm for contemporary nutrition? *Proc. Nutr. Soc.* 65, 1–6 (2006).

177. Wikipedia contributors. Dietary Fiber. *Wikipedia* (2016). Available at: https://en.wikipedia.org/w/index.php?title=Dietary_fiber&oldid=722234024. (Accessed: 31st May 2016)

178. Arslanoglu, S. et al. Early dietary intervention with a mixture of prebiotic oligosaccharides reduces the incidence of allergic manifestations and infections during the first two years of life. *J. Nutr.* 138, 1091–1095 (2008).

179. Ivakhnenko, O. S. & Nyankovskyy, S. L. Effect of the specific infant formula mixture of oligosaccharides on local immunity and development of allergic and infectious disease in young children: Randomized study. *Pediatr. Pol.* 88, 398–404 (2013).

180. Kondo, T., Kishi, M., Fushimi, T., Ugajin, S. & Kaga, T. Vinegar intake reduces body weight, body fat mass, and serum triglyceride levels in obese Japanese subjects. *Biosci. Biotechnol. Biochem.* 73, 1837–1843 (2009).

181. Thorburn, A. N. et al. Evidence that asthma is a developmental origin disease influenced by maternal diet and bacterial metabolites. *Nat. Commun.* 6, 7320 (2015).

182. King, D. E. et al. Effect of a high-fiber diet vs a fiber-supplemented diet on C-reactive protein level. *Arch. Intern. Med.* 167, 502–506 (2007).

183. Mayo Clinic Staff. Mediterranean Diet for Heart Health. *Mayo Clinic* (2016). Available at: http://www.mayoclinic.org/healthy-lifestyle/nutrition-and-healthy-eating/in-depth/mediterranean-diet/art-20047801. (Accessed: 4th June 2016)

184. Chatzi, L. et al. Mediterranean diet in pregnancy is protective for wheeze and atopy in childhood. *Thorax* 63, 507–513 (2008).

185. Rizkalla, S. W. et al. Chronic consumption of fresh but not heated yogurt improves breath-hydrogen status and short-chain fatty acid profiles: a controlled study in healthy men with or without lactose maldigestion1–3. *Am. J. Clin. Nutr.* 72, 1474–1479 (2000).

186. Roduit, C. et al. Development of atopic dermatitis according to age of onset and association with early-life exposures. *J. Allergy Clin. Immunol.* 130, 130–6.e5 (2012).

187. Shoda, T. et al. Yogurt consumption in infancy is inversely associated with atopic dermatitis and food sensitization at 5 years of age: A hospital-based birth cohort study. *J. Dermatol. Sci.* 86, 90–96 (2017).

188. Crane, J. et al. Is yoghurt an acceptable alternative to raw milk for reducing eczema and allergy in infancy? *Clin. Exp. Allergy* 48, 604–606 (2018).

189. Davis, N. Children's yoghurts contain "shocking" amounts of sugar, study finds. *The Guardian* (2018).

190. Rea, M. C. et al. Irish kefir-like grains: Their structure, microbial composition and fermentation kinetics. *J. Appl. Bacteriol.* **81**, 83–94 (1996).

191. Fu, C., Yan, F., Cao, Z., Xie, F. & Lin, J. Antioxidant activities of kombucha prepared from three different substrates and changes in content of probiotics during storage. *Food Sci. Technol.* **34**, 123–126 (2014).

192. Plengvidhya, V., Breidt, F., Jr, Lu, Z. & Fleming, H. P. DNA fingerprinting of lactic acid bacteria in sauerkraut fermentations. *Appl. Environ. Microbiol.* **73**, 7697–7702 (2007).

193. Lee, D., Kim, S., Cho, J. & Kim, J. Microbial population dynamics and temperature changes during fermentation of kimjang kimchi. *J. Microbiol.* **46**, 590–593 (2008).

194. Shewell, L. Everything you always wanted to know about fermented foods. *Science-Based Medicine* (2015). Available at: https://www.sciencebasedmedicine.org/everything-you-always-wanted-to-know-about-fermented-foods/#h.34godwd. (Accessed: 6th June 2016)

195. Heid, M. Experts Say Lobbying Skewed the U.S. Dietary Guidelines. *Time* (2016).

196. Nestle, M. Food lobbies, the food pyramid, and U.S. nutrition policy. *Int. J. Health Serv.* **23**, 483–496 (1993).

197. Press Association. Official advice on low-fat diet and cholesterol is wrong, says health charity. *The Guardian* (2016).

198. NIH, National Institute of General Medical Sciences (NIGMS). The biology of fats in the body. *ScienceDaily* (2013). Available at: https://www.sciencedaily.com/releases/2013/04/130423102127.htm. (Accessed: 13th June 2016)

199. Estruch, R. et al. Effect of a high-fat Mediterranean diet on bodyweight and waist circumference: A prespecified secondary outcomes analysis of the PREDIMED randomised controlled trial. *Lancet Diabetes Endocrinol* (2016). doi: 10.1016/S2213-8587(16)30085-7

200. Schwingshackl, L., Strasser, B. & Hoffmann, G. Effects of monounsaturated fatty acids on cardiovascular risk factors: A systematic review and meta-analysis. *Ann. Nutr. Metab.* **59**, 176–186 (2011).

201. McAuley, K. A. et al. Comparison of high-fat and high-protein diets with a high-carbohydrate diet in insulin-resistant obese women. *Diabetologia* **48**, 8–16 (2005).

202. Garg, A. High-monounsaturated-fat diets for patients with diabetes mellitus: A meta-analysis. *Am. J. Clin. Nutr.* **67**, 577S–582S (1998).

203. Simopoulos, A. P. Evolutionary Aspects of the Dietary Omega-6/Omega-3 Fatty Acid Ratio: Medical Implications. In *Evolutionary Thinking in Medicine* (eds. Alvergne, A., Jenkinson, C. & Faurie, C.) 119–134 (Springer International Publishing, 2016).

204. Mujico, J. R., Baccan, G. C., Gheorghe, A., Díaz, L. E. & Marcos, A. Changes in gut microbiota due to supplemented fatty acids in diet-induced obese mice. *Br. J. Nutr.* (2012). doi: 10.1017/S0007114512005612

205. Hidalgo, M. et al. Effect of virgin and refined olive oil consumption on gut microbiota. Comparison to butter. *Food Res. Int.* 64, 553–559 (2014).

206. Martín-Peláez, S., Covas, M. I., Fitó, M., Kušar, A. & Pravst, I. Health effects of olive oil polyphenols: Recent advances and possibilities for the use of health claims. *Mol. Nutr. Food Res.* 57, 760–771 (2013).

207. Schwingshackl, L. & Hoffmann, G. Monounsaturated fatty acids and risk of cardiovascular disease: Synopsis of the evidence available from systematic reviews and meta-analyses. *Nutrients* 4, 1989–2007 (2012).

208. Kris-Etherton, P. M. AHA Science Advisory. Monounsaturated fatty acids and risk of cardiovascular disease. American Heart Association. Nutrition Committee. *Circulation* 100, 1253–1258 (1999).

209. Menendez, J. A. & Lupu, R. Mediterranean dietary traditions for the molecular treatment of human cancer: Anti-oncogenic actions of the main olive oil's monounsaturated fatty acid oleic acid (18:1n-9). *Curr. Pharm. Biotechnol.* 7, 495–502 (2006).

210. Carrillo, C., Cavia, M. D. M. & Alonso-Torre, S. R. Antitumor effect of oleic acid; Mechanisms of action: A review. *Nutr. Hosp.* 27, 1860–1865 (2012).

211. Cicerale, S., Lucas, L. J. & Keast, R. S. J. Antimicrobial, antioxidant and anti-inflammatory phenolic activities in extra virgin olive oil. *Curr. Opin. Biotechnol.* 23, 129–135 (2012).

212. Lucas, L., Russell, A. & Keast, R. Molecular mechanisms of inflammation. Anti-inflammatory benefits of virgin olive oil and the phenolic compound oleocanthal. *Curr. Pharm. Des.* 17, 754–768 (2011).

213. Khalatbary, A. R. Olive oil phenols and neuroprotection. *Nutr. Neurosci.* 16, 243–249 (2013).

214. Bui-Klimke, T. R., Guclu, H., Kensler, T. W., Yuan, J.-M. & Wu, F. Aflatoxin regulations and global pistachio trade: Insights from social network analysis. *PLoS One* 9, e92149 (2014).

215. Commission of the European Communities. Commission Directive 80/891/EEC of 25 July 1980 relating to the community method of analysis for determining the erucic acid content in oils and fats intended to be used as such for human consumption and foodstuffs containing added oils or fats. (1980).

216. U.S. Food and Drug Administration. Code of Federal Regulations Title 21—Rapeseed Oil. (2015).

217. O'Keefe, S., Gaskins-Wright, S., Wiley, V. & Chen, I.-C. Levels of trans geometrical isomers of essential fatty acids in some unhydrogenated U. S. vegetable oils. *J. Food Lipids* 1, 165–176 (1994).

218. Davis, B. C. & Kris-Etherton, P. M. Achieving optimal essential fatty acid status in vegetarians: Current knowledge and practical implications. *Am. J. Clin. Nutr.* 78, 640S–646S (2003).

219. Li, B., Birdwell, C. & Whelan, J. Antithetic relationship of dietary arachidonic acid and eicosapentaenoic acid on eicosanoid production in vivo. *J. Lipid Res.* 35, 1869–1877 (1994).

220. Méndez-Salazar, E. O., Ortiz-López, M. G., Granados-Silvestre, M. de L. Á., Palacios-González, B. & Menjivar, M. Altered gut microbiota and compositional changes in firmicutes and proteobacteria in Mexican undernourished and obese children. *Front. Microbiol.* **9**, 2494 (2018).

221. Galipeau, H. J. et al. Intestinal microbiota modulates gluten-induced immunopathology in humanized mice. *Am. J. Pathol.* **185**, 2969–2982 (2015).

222. Ghosh, S. et al. Fish oil attenuates omega-6 polyunsaturated fatty acid-induced dysbiosis and infectious colitis but impairs LPS dephosphorylation activity causing sepsis. *PLoS One* **8**, e55468 (2013).

223. Hibbeln, J. R., Nieminen, L. R. G., Blasbalg, T. L., Riggs, J. A. & Lands, W. E. M. Healthy intakes of n-3 and n-6 fatty acids: Estimations considering worldwide diversity. *Am. J. Clin. Nutr.* **83**, 1483S–1493S (2006).

224. Hibbeln, J. R., Nieminen, L. R. G. & Lands, W. E. M. Increasing homicide rates and linoleic acid consumption among five western countries, 1961–2000. *Lipids* **39**, 1207–1213 (2004).

225. Kankaanpää, P. et al. Polyunsaturated fatty acids in maternal diet, breast milk, and serum lipid fatty acids of infants in relation to atopy. *Allergy* **56**, 633–638 (2001).

226. Sausenthaler, S. et al. Maternal diet during pregnancy in relation to eczema and allergic sensitization in the offspring at 2 y of age. *Am. J. Clin. Nutr.* **85**, 530–537 (2007).

227. Sausenthaler, S. et al. Margarine and butter consumption, eczema and allergic sensitization in children. The LISA birth cohort study. *Pediatr. Allergy Immunol.* **17**, 85–93 (2006).

228. Fitzsimon, N. et al. Mothers' dietary patterns during pregnancy and risk of asthma symptoms in children at 3 years. *Ir. Med. J.* **100**, suppl. 27–32 (2007).

229. Oddy, W. H. et al. Atopy, eczema and breast milk fatty acids in a high-risk cohort of children followed from birth to 5 yr. *Pediatr. Allergy Immunol.* **17**, 4–10 (2006).

230. Yang, L. G. et al. Low n-6/n-3 PUFA ratio improves lipid metabolism, inflammation, oxidative stress and endothelial function in rats using plant oils as n-3 fatty acid source. *Lipids* **51**, 49–59 (2016).

231. Simopoulos, A. P. The importance of the ratio of omega-6/omega-3 essential fatty acids. *Biomed. Pharmacother.* **56**, 365–379 (2002).

232. Lane, K., Derbyshire, E., Li, W. & Brennan, C. Bioavailability and potential uses of vegetarian sources of omega-3 fatty acids: A review of the literature. *Crit. Rev. Food Sci. Nutr.* **54**, 572–579 (2014).

233. Lee, H.-S. et al. Modulation of DNA methylation states and infant immune system by dietary supplementation with ω-3 PUFA during pregnancy in an intervention study. *Am. J. Clin. Nutr.* **98**, 480–487 (2013).

234. Gunaratne, A. W., Makrides, M. & Collins, C. T. Maternal prenatal and/or postnatal n-3 long chain polyunsaturated fatty acids (LCPUFA) supplementation for preventing allergies in early childhood. *Cochrane Database Syst. Rev.* **7**, CD010085 (2015).

235. Yang, H., Xun, P. & He, K. Fish and fish oil intake in relation to risk of asthma: A systematic review and meta-analysis. *PLoS One* **8**, e80048 (2013).

236. Oien, T., Storrø, O. & Johnsen, R. Do early intake of fish and fish oil protect against eczema and doctor-diagnosed asthma at 2 years of age? A cohort study. *J. Epidemiol. Community Health* **64**, 124–129 (2010).

237. Innis, S. M. Dietary (n-3) fatty acids and brain development. *J. Nutr.* **137**, 855–859 (2007).

238. Wu, A., Ying, Z. & Gomez-Pinilla, F. Docosahexaenoic acid dietary supplementation enhances the effects of exercise on synaptic plasticity and cognition. *Neuroscience* **155**, 751–759 (2008).

239. Hüppi, P. S. Nutrition for the brain: Commentary on the article by Isaacs et al. on page 308. *Pediatric research* **63**, 229–231 (2008).

240. Campoy, C., Escolano-Margarit, M. V., Anjos, T., Szajewska, H. & Uauy, R. Omega 3 fatty acids on child growth, visual acuity and neurodevelopment. *Br. J. Nutr.* **107** Suppl, S85–106 (2012).

241. Innis, S. M. Dietary omega 3 fatty acids and the developing brain. *Brain Res.* **1237**, 35–43 (2008).

242. Meng, Q. et al. Systems nutrigenomics reveals brain gene networks linking metabolic and brain disorders. *EBioMedicine* **7**, 157–166 (2016).

243. McNamara, R. K. & Carlson, S. E. Role of omega-3 fatty acids in brain development and function: Potential implications for the pathogenesis and prevention of psychopathology. *Prostaglandins Leukot. Essent. Fatty Acids* **75**, 329–349 (2006).

244. Lederman, S. A. et al. Relation between cord blood mercury levels and early child development in a World Trade Center cohort. *Environ. Health Perspect.* **116**, 1085–1091 (2008).

245. Hibbeln, J. R. et al. Maternal seafood consumption in pregnancy and neurodevelopmental outcomes in childhood (ALSPAC study): An observational cohort study. *Lancet* **369**, 578–585 (2007).

246. Scheer, R. & Moss, D. Harvest of Fears: Farm-Raised Fish May Not Be Free of Mercury and Other Pollutants. *Scientific American* (2016).

247. U.S. Food and Drug Administration. Metals—Mercury Levels in Commercial Fish and Shellfish (1990-2010). *FDA.gov* (2014). Available at: http://www.fda.gov/Food/FoodborneIllnessContaminants/Metals/ucm115644.htm. (Accessed: 6th November 2016)

248. Mayo Clinic Staff. Pregnancy and Fish: What's Safe to Eat?—Mayo Clinic. *Mayo Clinic* (2016). Available at: http://www.mayoclinic.org/healthy-lifestyle/pregnancy-week-by-week/in-depth/pregnancy-and-fish/art-20044185. (Accessed: 7th November 2016)

249. Sørmo, E. G. et al. Selenium moderates mercury toxicity in free-ranging freshwater fish. *Environ. Sci. Technol.* **45**, 6561–6566 (2011).

250. da Conceição Nascimento Pinheiro, M., do Nascimento, J. L. M., de Lima Silveira, L. C., da Rocha, J. B. T. & Aschner, M. Mercury and selenium—A review on aspects related to the health of human populations in the Amazon. *Environ. Bioindicators* 4, 222–245 (2009).

251. Ralston, N. V. C., Ralston, C. R., Blackwell, J. L., 3rd & Raymond, L. J. Dietary and tissue selenium in relation to methylmercury toxicity. *Neurotoxicology* 29, 802–811 (2008).

252. Kaneko, J. J. & Ralston, N. V. C. Selenium and mercury in pelagic fish in the central north pacific near Hawaii. *Biol. Trace Elem. Res.* 119, 242–254 (2007).

253. Burger, J., Jeitner, C. & Gochfeld, M. Locational differences in mercury and selenium levels in 19 species of saltwater fish from New Jersey. *J. Toxicol. Environ. Health A* 74, 863–874 (2011).

254. Global Organisation for EPA and DHA. *Global Recommendations for EPA and DHA Intake.* (International Society for the Study of Fatty Acids and Lipids, 2014).

255. Koletzko, B., Cetin, I. & Brenna, J. T. Dietary fat intakes for pregnant and lactating women. *British Journal of Nutrition* 98, 873–877 (2007).

256. Dietary Guidelines Advisory Committee. 2005 Dietary Guidelines Advisory Committee Report—Addendum A: EPA and DHA Content of Fish Species. *Health.gov* (2005). Available at: https://health.gov/dietaryguidelines/dga2005/report/html/table_g2_adda2. htm. (Accessed: 8th November 2016)

257. Good Fish Guide. *Marine Conservation Society* Available at: https://www.mcsuk.org/ goodfishguide/search. (Accessed: 20th May 2019)

258. Visioli, F., Risé, P., Barassi, M. C., Marangoni, F. & Galli, C. Dietary intake of fish vs. formulations leads to higher plasma concentrations of n-3 fatty acids. *Lipids* 38, 415–418 (2003).

259. Teicholz, N. The science of saturated fat: A big fat surprise about nutrition? *The Independent* (2014).

260. Chowdhury, R. et al. Association of dietary, circulating, and supplement fatty acids with coronary risk: A systematic review and meta-analysis. *Ann. Intern. Med.* 160, 398–406 (2014).

261. de Souza, R. J. et al. Intake of saturated and trans unsaturated fatty acids and risk of all cause mortality, cardiovascular disease, and type 2 diabetes: Systematic review and meta-analysis of observational studies. *BMJ* 351, h3978 (2015).

262. Bouvard, V. et al. Carcinogenicity of consumption of red and processed meat. *Lancet Oncol.* 16, 1599–1600 (2015).

263. Simon, S. World Health Organization Says Processed Meat Causes Cancer. *Cancer.org* (2015). Available at: http://www.cancer.org/cancer/news/news/world-health-organization-says-processed-meat-causes-cancer. (Accessed: 23rd June 2016)

264. World Health Organization. Q&A on the Carcinogenicity of the Consumption of Red Meat and Processed Meat. (2015). Available at: http://www.who.int/features/qa/cancer-red-meat/ en/. (Accessed: 23rd June 2016)

265. Samraj, A. N. et al. A red meat-derived glycan promotes inflammation and cancer progression. *Proc. Natl. Acad. Sci. U. S. A.* 112, 542–547 (2015).

266. Gratz, S. W. Balancing Dietary Fibre and Protein for a Healthy Gut. *The Nutrition Society* (2013). Available at: https://www.nutritionsociety.org/yournutrition/articles/balancing-dietary-fibre-and-protein-healthy-gut. (Accessed: 23rd June 2016)

267. Holtrop, G., Johnstone, A. M., Fyfe, C. & Gratz, S. W. Diet composition is associated with endogenous formation of N-nitroso compounds in obese men. *J. Nutr.* 142, 1652–1658 (2012).

268. Larsson, S. C., Bergkvist, L. & Wolk, A. Milk and lactose intakes and ovarian cancer risk in the Swedish Mammography Cohort1-3. *Am. J. Clin. Nutr.* 80, 1353–1357 (2004).

269. Barnard, N. D. *Milk Consumption and Prostate Cancer.* (Physicians Committee for Responsible Medicine, 2015).

270. Kroenke, C. H., Kwan, M. L., Sweeney, C., Castillo, A. & Caan, B. J. High- and low-fat dairy intake, recurrence, and mortality after breast cancer diagnosis. *J. Natl. Cancer Inst.* 105, 616–623 (2013).

271. Holmes, M. D., Pollak, M. N., Willett, W. C. & Hankinson, S. E. Dietary correlates of plasma insulin-like growth factor I and insulin-like growth factor binding protein 3 concentrations. *Cancer Epidemiol. Biomarkers Prev.* 11, 852–861 (2002).

272. Grimberg, A. Mechanisms by which IGF-I may promote cancer. *Cancer Biol. Ther.* 2, 630–635 (2003).

273. Weroha, S. J. & Haluska, P. The insulin-like growth factor system in cancer. *Endocrinol. Metab. Clin. North Am.* 41, 335–50, vi (2012).

274. Romo Ventura, E. et al. Association of dietary intake of milk and dairy products with blood concentrations of insulin-like growth factor 1 (IGF-1) in Bavarian adults. *Eur. J. Nutr.* (2019). doi: 10.1007/s00394-019-01994-7

275. Kang, S. H., Kim, J. U., Imm, J. Y., Oh, S. & Kim, S. H. The effects of dairy processes and storage on insulin-like growth factor-I (IGF-I) content in milk and in model IGF-I-fortified dairy products. *J. Dairy Sci.* 89, 402–409 (2006).

276. Daxenberger, A., Breier, B. H. & Sauerwein, H. Increased milk levels of insulin-like growth factor 1 (IGF-1) for the identification of bovine somatotropin (bST) treated cows. *Analyst* 123, 2429–2435 (1998).

277. Shen, W., Gaskins, H. R. & McIntosh, M. K. Influence of dietary fat on intestinal microbes, inflammation, barrier function and metabolic outcomes. *J. Nutr. Biochem.* 25, 270–280 (2014).

278. Caesar, R., Tremaroli, V., Kovatcheva-Datchary, P., Cani, P. D. & Bäckhed, F. Crosstalk between gut microbiota and dietary lipids aggravates WAT inflammation through TLR Signaling. *Cell Metab.* (2015). doi: 10.1016/j.cmet.2015.07.026

279. Devkota, S. et al. Dietary-fat-induced taurocholic acid promotes pathobiont expansion and colitis in Il10-/- mice. *Nature* 487, 104–108 (2012).

280. Harmon, K. Saturated Fats Change Gut Bacteria and May Raise Risk for Inflammatory Bowel Disease. *Scientific American* (2012). Available at: http://blogs.scientificamerican.com/ observations/saturated-fats-change-gut-bacteria-and-may-raise-risk-for-inflammatory-bowel-disease/. (Accessed: 15th June 2016)

281. Myles, I. A. Fast food fever: Reviewing the impacts of the western diet on immunity. *Nutr. J.* 13, 61 (2014).

282. Yandell, K. How Fats Influence the Microbiome. *The Scientist* (2015). Available at: http:// www.the-scientist.com/?articles.view/articleNo/43854/title/How-Fats-Influence-the-Microbiome/. (Accessed: 15th June 2016)

283. Laugerette, F. et al. Oil composition of high-fat diet affects metabolic inflammation differently in connection with endotoxin receptors in mice. *Am. J. Physiol. Endocrinol. Metab.* 302, E374–86 (2012).

284. Kabagambe, E. K., Baylin, A., Ascherio, A. & Campos, H. The type of oil used for cooking is associated with the risk of nonfatal acute myocardial infarction in Costa Rica. *J. Nutr.* 135, 2674–2679 (2005).

285. Joshi-Barve, S. et al. Palmitic acid induces production of proinflammatory cytokine interleukin-8 from hepatocytes. *Hepatology* 46, 823–830 (2007).

286. Milman, O. Palm oil labelling in Australia could become a reality if bill passes. *The Guardian* (2011).

287. Rival, A. & Levang, P. *Palms of controversies: Oil palm and development challenges.* (Center for International Forestry Research, 2014). doi: 10.17528/cifor/004860

288. Intahphuak, S., Khonsung, P. & Panthong, A. Anti-inflammatory, analgesic, and antipyretic activities of virgin coconut oil. *Pharm. Biol.* 48, 151–157 (2010).

289. Zakaria, Z. A. et al. In vivo antinociceptive and anti-inflammatory activities of dried and fermented processed virgin coconut oil. *Med. Princ. Pract.* 20, 231–236 (2011).

290. Peedikayil, F. C., Sreenivasan, P. & Narayanan, A. Effect of coconut oil in plaque related gingivitis—a preliminary report. *Niger. Med. J.* 56, 143–147 (2015).

291. Kamisah, Y. et al. Cardioprotective effect of virgin coconut oil in heated palm oil diet-induced hypertensive rats. *Pharm. Biol.* 53, 1243–1249 (2015).

292. Eyres, L., Eyres, M. F., Chisholm, A. & Brown, R. C. Coconut oil consumption and cardiovascular risk factors in humans. *Nutr. Rev.* 74, 267–280 (2016).

293. Khaw, K.-T. et al. Randomised trial of coconut oil, olive oil or butter on blood lipids and other cardiovascular risk factors in healthy men and women. *BMJ Open* 8, e020167 (2018).

294. Palazhy, S., Kamath, P. & Vasudevan, D. M. dietary fats and oxidative stress: A cross-sectional study among coronary artery disease subjects consuming coconut oil/sunflower oil. *Indian J. Clin. Biochem.* 33, 69–74 (2018).

295. Vijayakumar, M. et al. A randomized study of coconut oil versus sunflower oil on cardiovascular risk factors in patients with stable coronary heart disease. *Indian Heart J.* 68, 498–506 (2016).

296. Mozaffarian, D., Katan, M. B., Ascherio, A., Stampfer, M. J. & Willett, W. C. Trans fatty acids and cardiovascular disease. *N. Engl. J. Med.* 354, 1601–1613 (2006).

297. Belluz, J. & Collins, D. The New Global Plan to Eliminate the Most Harmful Fat in food, explained. *Vox* (2018). Available at: https://www.vox.com/science-and-health/2018/5/14/17346108/trans-fats-food-world-health-organization-bloomberg-gates. (Accessed: 13th May 2019)

298. U.S. Food & Drug Administration. Final Determination Regarding Partially Hydrogenated Oils. *FDA.gov* (2018). Available at: https://www.fda.gov/food/food-additives-petitions/final-determination-regarding-partially-hydrogenated-oils-removing-trans-fat. (Accessed: 13th May 2019)

299. Food and Drug Administration. Final Determination Regarding Partially Hydrogenated Oils. *Federal Register* (2015). Available at: https://www.federalregister.gov/articles/2015/06/17/2015-14883/final-determination-regarding-partially-hydrogenated-oils. (Accessed: 22nd July 2016)

300. Lindmeier, C. & Lawe Davies, O. WHO Calls on Countries to Reduce Sugars Intake among Adults and Children. *World Health Organization* (2015). Available at: https://www.who.int/mediacentre/news/releases/2015/sugar-guideline/en/. (Accessed: 4th November 2019)

301. Herrick, K. Consumption of added sugars among U.S. infants aged 6–23 months, 2011–2014. In *Nutrition 2018* (American Society for Nutrition, 2018).

302. BBC News—Health. Sugar Intake in Children "Double Recommended Level." *BBC* (2016). Available at: http://www.bbc.com/news/health-37318193. (Accessed: 27th January 2017)

303. Williams, Z. Robert Lustig: The man who believes sugar is poison. *The Guardian* (2014).

304. World Health Organization. Obesity and Overweight. (2016).

305. Hackethal, V. Type 2 Diabetes Rates Quadruple Worldwide since 1980. *Medscape* (2016). Available at: http://www.medscape.com/viewarticle/861591. (Accessed: 27th January 2017)

306. Sanchez, A. et al. Role of sugars in human neutrophilic phagocytosis. *Am. J. Clin. Nutr.* 26, 1180–1184 (1973).

307. Jameel, F., Phang, M., Wood, L. G. & Garg, M. L. Acute effects of feeding fructose, glucose and sucrose on blood lipid levels and systemic inflammation. *Lipids Health Dis.* 13, 195 (2014).

308. Esposito, K. et al. Inflammatory cytokine concentrations are acutely increased by hyperglycemia in humans: Role of oxidative stress. *Circulation* 106, 2067–2072 (2002).

309. Stanhope, K. L., Schwarz, J.-M. & Havel, P. J. Adverse metabolic effects of dietary fructose: Results from the recent epidemiological, clinical, and mechanistic studies. *Curr. Opin. Lipidol.* 24, 198–206 (2013).

310. Bray, G. A. How bad is fructose? *Am. J. Clin. Nutr.* 86, 895–896 (2007).

311. Leech, J. Agave Nectar: A Sweetener That Is Even Worse Than Sugar. *Authority Nutrition* (2014). Available at: https://authoritynutrition.com/agave-nectar-is-even-worse-than-sugar/. (Accessed: 15th March 2017)

312. Gunnars, K. Fruit Juice Is Just as Unhealthy as a Sugary Drink. *Authority Nutrition* (2014). Available at: https://authoritynutrition.com/fruit-juice-is-just-as-bad-as-soda/. (Accessed: 15th March 2017)

313. Brown, K., DeCoffe, D., Molcan, E. & Gibson, D. L. Diet-induced dysbiosis of the intestinal microbiota and the effects on immunity and disease. *Nutrients* 4, 1095–1119 (2012).

314. Crook, W. G. Vaginal yeast infections exacerbated by sugar intake. *The Nurse Practitioner* 18, 8 (1993).

315. Penders, J. et al. Molecular fingerprinting of the intestinal microbiota of infants in whom atopic eczema was or was not developing. *Clin. Exp. Allergy* 36, 1602–1608 (2006).

316. Akinbi, H. T., Narendran, V., Pass, A. K., Markart, P. & Hoath, S. B. Host defense proteins in vernix caseosa and amniotic fluid. *American Journal of Obstetrics and Gynecology* 191, 2090–2096 (2004).

317. Bédard, A., Northstone, K., Henderson, A. J. & Shaheen, S. O. Maternal intake of sugar during pregnancy and childhood respiratory and atopic outcomes. *Eur. Respir. J.* 50, (2017).

318. Manzel, A. et al. Role of "western diet" in inflammatory autoimmune diseases. *Curr. Allergy Asthma Rep.* 14, 404 (2014).

319. Yong, E. Fat Cell Number Is Set in Childhood and Stays Constant in Adulthood. *Not Exactly Rocket Science* (2008). Available at: http://scienceblogs.com/notrocketscience/2008/05/04/fat-cell-number-is-set-in-childhood-and-stays-constant-in-ad/. (Accessed: 16th March 2017)

320. Callahan, A. Are Fat Cells Forever? *The New York Times* (2017).

321. Gifford, B. Your Fat Has a Brain. Seriously. And It's Trying to Kill You. *Outside Online* (2013). Available at: https://www.outsideonline.com/1914196/your-fat-has-brain-seriously-and-its-trying-kill-you. (Accessed: 16th March 2017)

322. Chu, S. Y. et al. Maternal obesity and risk of gestational diabetes mellitus. *Diabetes Care* 30, 2070–2076 (2007).

323. Ferrara, A. Increasing prevalence of gestational diabetes mellitus: A public health perspective. *Diabetes Care* 30 **Suppl 2,** S141–6 (2007).

324. The HAPO Study Cooperative Research Group. Hyperglycemia and adverse pregnancy outcomes. *N. Engl. J. Med.* 358, 1991–2002 (2008).

325. Center for Vulnerable Populations at San Francisco General Hospital and Trauma Center. *Issue Brief: Chronic Disease Risk—Gestational Diabetes.* (University of California San Francisco, 2013).

326. Kumar, R. et al. Gestational diabetes, atopic dermatitis, and allergen sensitization in early childhood. *J. Allergy Clin. Immunol.* 124, 1031–8.e1–4 (2009).

327. Eteraf-Oskouei, T. & Najafi, M. Traditional and modern uses of natural honey in human diseases: A review. *Iran. J. Basic Med. Sci.* 16, 731–742 (2013).

328. Al-Waili, N. S. Natural honey lowers plasma glucose, C-reactive protein, homocysteine, and blood lipids in healthy, diabetic, and hyperlipidemic subjects: Comparison with dextrose and sucrose. *J. Med. Food* 7, 100–107 (2004).

329. Yaghoobi, N. et al. Natural honey and cardiovascular risk factors: Effects on blood glucose, cholesterol, triacylglycerole, CRP, and body weight compared with sucrose. *Scientific World Journal* 8, 463–469 (2008).

330. Abdulrhman, M. M. et al. Metabolic effects of honey in type 1 diabetes mellitus: A randomized crossover pilot study. *J. Med. Food* 16, 66–72 (2013).

331. Bahrami, M. et al. Effects of natural honey consumption in diabetic patients: An 8-week randomized clinical trial. *Int. J. Food Sci. Nutr.* 60, 618–626 (2009).

332. Al-Waili, N. S. & Boni, N. S. Natural honey lowers plasma prostaglandin concentrations in normal individuals. *J. Med. Food* 6, 129–133 (2003).

333. Porcza, L., Simms, C. & Chopra, M. Honey and cancer: Current status and future directions. *Diseases* 4, 30 (2016).

334. Ahmed, S. & Othman, N. H. Honey as a potential natural anticancer agent: A review of its mechanisms. *Evid. Based. Complement. Alternat. Med.* 2013, 829070 (2013).

335. Li, L. & Seeram, N. P. Further investigation into maple syrup yields 3 new lignans, a new phenylpropanoid, and 26 other phytochemicals. *J. Agric. Food Chem.* 59, 7708–7716 (2011).

336. Abou-Zaid, M. M., Nozzolillo, C., Tonon, A., Coppens, M. & Lombardo, D. A. High-performance liquid chromatography characterization and identification of antioxidant polyphenols in maple syrup. *Pharm. Biol.* 46, 117–125 (2008).

337. Yamamoto, T., Uemura, K., Moriyama, K., Mitamura, K. & Taga, A. Inhibitory effect of maple syrup on the cell growth and invasion of human colorectal cancer cells. *Oncol. Rep.* 33, 1579–1584 (2015).

338. González-Sarrías, A., Ma, H., Edmonds, M. E. & Seeram, N. P. Maple polyphenols, ginnalins A–C, induce S- and G2/M-cell cycle arrest in colon and breast cancer cells mediated by decreasing cyclins A and D1 levels. *Food Chem.* 136, 636–642 (2013).

339. González-Sarrías, A., Li, L. & Seeram, N. P. Effects of maple (Acer) plant part extracts on proliferation, apoptosis and cell cycle arrest of human tumorigenic and non-tumorigenic colon cells. *Phytother. Res.* 26, 995–1002 (2012).

340. Yang, Q. Gain weight by "going diet"? Artificial sweeteners and the neurobiology of sugar cravings: Neuroscience 2010. *Yale J. Biol. Med.* 83, 101–108 (2010).

341. Pepino, M. Y. Metabolic effects of non-nutritive sweeteners. *Physiol. Behav.* 152, 450–455 (2015).

342. Just, T., Pau, H. W., Engel, U. & Hummel, T. Cephalic phase insulin release in healthy humans after taste stimulation? *Appetite* 51, 622–627 (2008).

343. Suez, J. et al. Artificial sweeteners induce glucose intolerance by altering the gut microbiota. *Nature* 514, 181–186 (2014).

344. Suez, J., Korem, T., Zilberman-Schapira, G., Segal, E. & Elinav, E. Non-caloric artificial sweeteners and the microbiome: Findings and challenges. *Gut Microbes* 6, 149–155 (2015).

345. Velasquez-Manoff, M. The Germs That Love Diet Soda. *The New York Times* (2018).

346. Trasande, L., Shaffer, R. M., Sathyanarayana, S. & Council on Environmental Health. Food additives and child health. *Pediatrics* 142 (2018).

347. McBride, D. L. Safety concerns about food additives and children's health. *J. Pediatr. Nurs.* 45, 76–77 (2019).

348. Marion-Letellier, R., Amamou, A., Savoye, G. & Ghosh, S. Inflammatory bowel diseases and food additives: To add fuel on the flames! *Nutrients* 11 (2019).

349. Collins, J. et al. Dietary trehalose enhances virulence of epidemic *Clostridium difficile*. *Nature* 553, 291–294 (2018).

350. Nickerson, K. P. & McDonald, C. Crohn's disease-associated adherent-invasive *Escherichia coli* adhesion is enhanced by exposure to the ubiquitous dietary polysaccharide maltodextrin. *PLoS One* 7, e52132 (2012).

351. University of Bonn. Fast food makes the immune system more aggressive in the long term: Study shows that even after a change to a healthy diet, the body's defenses remain hyperactive. *Science Daily* (2018).

352. Christ, A. et al. Western diet triggers NLRP3-dependent innate immune reprogramming. *Cell* 172, 162–175.e14 (2018).

353. Kim, Y., Keogh, J. B. & Clifton, P. M. Polyphenols and glycemic control. *Nutrients* 8 (2016).

354. Mcdougall, G. J. & Stewart, D. The inhibitory effects of berry polyphenols on digestive enzymes. *Biofactors* 23, 189–195 (2005).

355. Bernardo, M. A. et al. Effect of cinnamon tea on postprandial glucose concentration. *Journal of Diabetes Research* 2015, 913651 (2015).

356. Hepper, P. Unravelling our beginnings. *Psychologist* 18, 474–477 (2005).

357. Fleming, A. How a child's food preferences begin in the womb. *The Guardian* (2014).

358. Mennella, J. A. Ontogeny of taste preferences: Basic biology and implications for health. *Am. J. Clin. Nutr.* 99, 704S–11S (2014).

359. Bayol, S. A., Farrington, S. J. & Stickland, N. C. A maternal "junk food" diet in pregnancy and lactation promotes an exacerbated taste for "junk food" and a greater propensity for obesity in rat offspring. *Br. J. Nutr.* 98, 843–851 (2007).

360. Patelarou, E. et al. Association between biomarker-quantified antioxidant status during pregnancy and infancy and allergic disease during early childhood: A systematic review. *Nutr. Rev.* 69, 627–641 (2011).

361. Nurmatov, U., Devereux, G. & Sheikh, A. Nutrients and foods for the primary prevention of asthma and allergy: Systematic review and meta-analysis. *J. Allergy Clin. Immunol.* 127, 724–33.e1–30 (2011).

362. Collier, J. Storage of Micronutrients in the Body. *Dietetics* (2008). Available at: http://www. dietetics.co.uk/micronutrient-storage.aspx. (Accessed: 1st May 2017)

363. King, J. C. The risk of maternal nutritional depletion and poor outcomes increases in early or closely spaced pregnancies. *J. Nutr.* 133, 1732S–1736S (2003).

364. Green, N. S. Folic acid supplementation and prevention of birth defects. *J. Nutr.* 132, 2356S–2360S (2002).

365. Viswanathan, M. et al. Folic acid supplementation for the prevention of neural tube defects: An updated evidence report and systematic review for the US Preventive Services Task Force. *JAMA* 317, 190–203 (2017).

366. Julvez, J. et al. Maternal use of folic acid supplements during pregnancy and four-year-old neurodevelopment in a population-based birth cohort. *Paediatr. Perinat. Epidemiol.* 23, 199–206 (2009).

367. Schlotz, W. et al. Lower maternal folate status in early pregnancy is associated with childhood hyperactivity and peer problems in offspring. *J. Child Psychol. Psychiatry* 51, 594–602 (2010).

368. Deloughery, T. G. et al. Common mutation in methylenetetrahydrofolate reductase. Correlation with homocysteine metabolism and late-onset vascular disease. *Circulation* 94, 3074–3078 (1996).

369. Ledowsky, C. The Folic Acid vs 5-MTHF Debate. *MTHFR Support* (2015). Available at: https://www.mthfrsupport.com.au/folic-acid-vs-5-mthf-debate/.

370. Leech, J. L-Methylfolate (5-MTHF): Your Must-Read Beginner's Guide. *DIET vs DISEASE* (2016). Available at: https://www.dietvsdisease.org/l-methylfolate-5-mthf/. (Accessed: 22nd June 2017)

371. Chavarro, J. E., Rich-Edwards, J. W., Rosner, B. A. & Willett, W. C. Use of multivitamins, intake of B vitamins, and risk of ovulatory infertility. *Fertil. Steril.* 89, 668–676 (2008).

372. The Natural Standard Research Collaboration. Folate—Safety. *Mayo Clinic* (2014). Available at: http://www.mayoclinic.org/drugs-supplements/folate/safety/hrb-20059475. (Accessed: 23rd June 2017)

373. Weiss, S. T. & Litonjua, A. A. Maternal diet vs lack of exposure to sunlight as the cause of the epidemic of asthma, allergies and other autoimmune diseases. *Thorax* 62, 746–748 (2007).

374. Aranow, C. Vitamin D and the immune system. *J. Investig. Med.* 59, 881–886 (2011).

375. Aghajafari, F. et al. Association between maternal serum 25-hydroxyvitamin D level and pregnancy and neonatal outcomes: Systematic review and meta-analysis of observational studies. *BMJ* 346, f1169 (2013).

376. Martineau, A. R. et al. Vitamin D for the management of asthma. *Cochrane Database Syst. Rev.* 9, CD011511 (2016).

377. Litonjua, A. A. Vitamin D deficiency as a risk factor for childhood allergic disease and asthma. *Curr. Opin. Allergy Clin. Immunol.* 12, 179–185 (2012).

378. Comberiati, P. et al. Is vitamin D deficiency correlated with childhood wheezing and asthma? *Front. Biosci.* **6**, 31–39 (2014).

379. Kolokotroni, O., Middleton, N., Kouta, C., Raftopoulos, V. & Yiallouros, P. K. Association of serum vitamin d with asthma and atopy in childhood: Review of epidemiological observational studies. *Mini Rev. Med. Chem.* **15**, 881–899 (2015).

380. Miyake, Y., Sasaki, S., Tanaka, K. & Hirota, Y. Dairy food, calcium and vitamin D intake in pregnancy, and wheeze and eczema in infants. *Eur. Respir. J.* **35**, 1228–1234 (2010).

381. Chawes, B. L. et al. Cord blood 25(OH)-vitamin D deficiency and childhood asthma, allergy and eczema: The COPSAC2000 birth cohort study. *PLoS One* **9**, e99856 (2014).

382. Gazibara, T. et al. Associations of maternal and fetal 25-hydroxyvitamin D levels with childhood eczema: The Generation R study. *Pediatr. Allergy Immunol.* **27**, 283–289 (2016).

383. Veugelers, P. & Ekwaru, J. A statistical error in the estimation of the recommended dietary allowance for vitamin D. *Nutrients* **6**, 4472–4475 (2014).

384. Creighton University. Recommendation for Vitamin D Intake Was Miscalculated, Is Far Too Low, Experts Say. *ScienceDaily* (2015). Available at: https://www.sciencedaily.com/releases/2015/03/150317122458.htm. (Accessed: 31st July 2017)

385. Roth, D. E. Vitamin D supplementation during pregnancy: Safety considerations in the design and interpretation of clinical trials. *J. Perinatol.* **31**, 449–459 (2011).

386. Cannell, J. J., Hollis, B. W., Zasloff, M. & Heaney, R. P. Diagnosis and treatment of vitamin D deficiency. *Expert Opin. Pharmacother.* **9**, 107–118 (2008)

387. Georgieff, M. K. The role of iron in neurodevelopment: Fetal iron deficiency and the developing hippocampus. *Biochem. Soc. Trans.* **36**, 1267–1271 (2008).

388. Nwaru, B. I. et al. An exploratory study of the associations between maternal iron status in pregnancy and childhood wheeze and atopy. *Br. J. Nutr.* **112**, 2018–2027 (2014).

389. Beard, J. Iron deficiency alters brain development and functioning. *J. Nutr.* **133**, 1468S–72S (2003).

390. Radlowski, E. C. & Johnson, R. W. Perinatal iron deficiency and neurocognitive development. *Front. Hum. Neurosci.* **7**, 585 (2013).

391. Lozoff, B. et al. Long-lasting neural and behavioral effects of iron deficiency in infancy. *Nutr. Rev.* **64**, S34–43; discussion S72–91 (2006).

392. NIH Office of Dietary Supplements. Iron—Fact Sheet. *National Institutes of Health* (2016). Available at: https://ods.od.nih.gov/factsheets/Iron-HealthProfessional/. (Accessed: 1st August 2017)

393. Fidler, M. C., Davidsson, L., Zeder, C. & Hurrell, R. F. Erythorbic acid is a potent enhancer of nonheme-iron absorption. *Am. J. Clin. Nutr.* **79**, 99–102 (2004).

394. Lönnerdal, B. Calcium and iron absorption—mechanisms and public health relevance. *Int. J. Vitam. Nutr. Res.* **80**, 293–299 (2010).

395. World's Healthiest Foods Staff. Iron. *World's Healthiest Foods* (2017). Available at: http://www.whfoods.com/genpage.php?tname=nutrient&dbid=70. (Accessed: 1st August 2017)

396. Caulfield, L. E. & Black, R. E. Zinc deficiency. In *Comparative Quantification of Health Risks* (eds. Ezzati, M., Lopez, A. D., Rodgers, A. & Murray, C. J. L.) 257–279 (World Health Organization, 2004).

397. Devereux, G. et al. Low maternal vitamin e intake during pregnancy is associated with asthma in 5-year-old children. *Am. J. Respir. Crit. Care Med.* 174, 499–507 (2006).

398. Litonjua, A. A. et al. Maternal antioxidant intake in pregnancy and wheezing illnesses in children at 2 y of age. *Am. J. Clin. Nutr.* 84, 903–911 (2006).

399. NIH Office of Dietary Supplements. Iodine—Fact Sheet. *National Institutes of Health* (2016). Available at: https://ods.od.nih.gov/factsheets/Iodine-Consumer/. (Accessed: 8th August 2017)

400. Brady, B. Thyroid Gland, How It Functions, Symptoms of Hyperthyroidism and Hypothyroidism. *EndocrineWeb* (2017). Available at: https://www.endocrineweb.com/conditions/thyroid-nodules/thyroid-gland-controls-bodys-metabolism-how-it-works-symptoms-hyperthyroi. (Accessed: 8th August 2017)

401. Hollowell, J. G. & Haddow, J. E. The prevalence of iodine deficiency in women of reproductive age in the United States of America. *Public Health Nutr.* 10, 1532–1539; discussion 1540–1541 (2007).

402. Morse, N. L. Benefits of docosahexaenoic acid, folic acid, vitamin D and iodine on foetal and infant brain development and function following maternal supplementation during pregnancy and lactation. *Nutrients* 4, 799–840 (2012).

403. Marques, A. H., O'Connor, T. G., Roth, C., Susser, E. & Bjørke-Monsen, A.-L. The influence of maternal prenatal and early childhood nutrition and maternal prenatal stress on offspring immune system development and neurodevelopmental disorders. *Front. Neurosci.* 7, 120 (2013).

404. World's Healthiest Foods Staff. Iodine. *World's Healthiest Foods* (2017). Available at: http://www.whfoods.com/genpage.php?tname=nutrient&dbid=69. (Accessed: 9th August 2017)

405. Weigel, R. M. & Weigel, M. M. Nausea and vomiting of early pregnancy and pregnancy outcome. A meta-analytical review. *Br. J. Obstet. Gynaecol.* 96, 1312–1318 (1989).

406. Forbes, S. Embryo quality: The missing link between pregnancy sickness and pregnancy outcome. *Evol. Hum. Behav.* 38, 265–278 (2017).

407. Jensen, H. H., Batres-Marquez, S. P., Carriquiry, A. & Schalinske, K. L. Choline in the diets of the US population: NHANES, 2003–2004. *FASEB J.* 21, LB46-c-(2007).

408. NIH Office of Dietary Supplements. Choline—Fact Sheet. *National Institutes of Health* (2017). Available at: https://ods.od.nih.gov/factsheets/Choline-HealthProfessional/. (Accessed: 10th August 2017)

409. Zeisel, S. H. Choline: Critical role during fetal development and dietary requirements in adults. *Annu. Rev. Nutr.* 26, 229–250 (2006).

410. Zeisel, S. H. The fetal origins of memory: The role of dietary choline in optimal brain development. *J. Pediatr.* 149, S131–6 (2006).

411. World's Healthiest Foods Staff. Choline. *World's Healthiest Foods* (2017). Available at: http://www.whfoods.com/genpage.php?tname=nutrient&dbid=50. (Accessed: 10th August 2017)

412. Troesch, B., Hoeft, B., McBurney, M., Eggersdorfer, M. & Weber, P. Dietary surveys indicate vitamin intakes below recommendations are common in representative western countries. *Br. J. Nutr.* 108, 692–698 (2012).

413. Péter, S. et al. A systematic review of global alpha-tocopherol status as assessed by nutritional intake levels and blood serum concentrations. *Int. J. Vitam. Nutr. Res.* 1–21 (2016).

414. McBurney, M. I. et al. Suboptimal serum α-tocopherol concentrations observed among younger adults and those depending exclusively upon food sources, NHANES 2003–2006. *PLoS One* 10, e0135510 (2015).

415. NIH Office of Dietary Supplements. Vitamin E—Fact Sheet. *National Institutes of Health* (2016). Available at: https://ods.od.nih.gov/factsheets/VitaminE-HealthProfessional/. (Accessed: 16th August 2017)

416. World's Healthiest Foods Staff. Vitamin E. *World's Healthiest Foods* (2017). Available at: http://www.whfoods.com/genpage.php?tname=nutrient&dbid=111. (Accessed: 16th August 2017)

417. Mansfield, J. A., Bergin, S. W., Cooper, J. R. & Olsen, C. H. Comparative probiotic strain efficacy in the prevention of eczema in infants and children: A systematic review and meta-analysis. *Mil. Med.* 179, 580–592 (2014).

418. Enomoto, T. et al. Effects of Bifidobacterial Supplementation to Pregnant Women and Infants in the Prevention of Allergy Development in Infants and on Fecal Microbiota. *Allergol. Int.* (2014). doi: 10.2332/allergolint.13-OA-0683

419. Elazab, N. et al. Probiotic administration in early life, atopy, and asthma: A meta-analysis of clinical trials. *Pediatrics* 132, e666–76 (2013).

420. Kuitunen, M. et al. Probiotics prevent IgE-associated allergy until age 5 years in cesarean-delivered children but not in the total cohort. *J. Allergy Clin. Immunol.* 123, 335–341 (2009).

421. Tang, M. L. K. et al. Administration of a probiotic with peanut oral immunotherapy: A randomized trial. *J. Allergy Clin. Immunol.* 135, 737–44.e8 (2015).

422. Hsiao, K.-C. et al. Long-term clinical and immunological effects of probiotic and peanut oral immunotherapy after treatment cessation: 4-year follow-up of a randomised, double-blind, placebo-controlled trial. *The Lancet Child & Adolescent Health* (2017). doi: 10.1016/S2352-4642(17)30041-X

423. Berni Canani, R. et al. Effect of *Lactobacillus* GG on tolerance acquisition in infants with cow's milk allergy: A randomized trial. *J. Allergy Clin. Immunol.* 129, 580–2, 582.e1–5 (2012).

424. Chen, Y.-S., Jan, R.-L., Lin, Y.-L., Chen, H.-H. & Wang, J.-Y. Randomized placebo-controlled trial of lactobacillus on asthmatic children with allergic rhinitis. *Pediatr. Pulmonol.* 45, 1111–1120 (2010).

425. Das, R. R., Naik, S. S. & Singh, M. Probiotics as additives on therapy in allergic airway diseases: A systematic review of benefits and risks. *Biomed Res. Int.* 2013, 231979 (2013).

426. Zajac, A. E., Adams, A. S. & Turner, J. H. A systematic review and meta-analysis of probiotics for the treatment of allergic rhinitis. *Int. Forum Allergy Rhinol.* 5, 524–532 (2015).

427. van der Aa, L. B. et al. Synbiotics prevent asthma-like symptoms in infants with atopic dermatitis. *Allergy* 66, 170–177 (2011).

428. Jang, S.-O. et al. Asthma prevention by *Lactobacillus rhamnosus* in a mouse model is associated with CD4(+)CD25(+)Foxp3(+) T cells. *Allergy Asthma Immunol. Res.* 4, 150–156 (2012).

429. Azad, M. B. et al. Probiotic supplementation during pregnancy or infancy for the prevention of asthma and wheeze: Systematic review and meta-analysis. *BMJ* 347, f6471 (2013).

430. Cabana, M. D. No consistent evidence to date that prenatal or postnatal probiotic supplementation prevents childhood asthma and wheeze. *Evidence-Based Medicine* 19, 144 (2014).

431. Laitinen, K., Poussa, T. & Isolauri, E. Probiotics and dietary counselling contribute to glucose regulation during and after pregnancy: A randomised controlled trial. *Br. J. Nutr.* 101, 1679–1687 (2009).

432. Brantsaeter, A. L. et al. Intake of probiotic food and risk of preeclampsia in primiparous women: The Norwegian Mother and Child cohort study. *Am. J. Epidemiol.* 174, 807–815 (2011).

433. Myhre, R. et al. Intake of probiotic food and risk of spontaneous preterm delivery. *Am. J. Clin. Nutr.* 93, 151–157 (2011).

434. Hao, Q., Dong, B. R. & Wu, T. Probiotics for preventing acute upper respiratory tract infections. *Cochrane Database Syst. Rev.* CD006895 (2015).

435. Skonieczna-Żydecka, K. et al. A systematic review, meta-analysis, and meta-regression evaluating the efficacy and mechanisms of action of probiotics and synbiotics in the prevention of surgical site infections and surgery-related complications. *J. Clin. Med. Res.* 7 (2018).

436. Kidd, P. M. Omega-3 DHA and EPA for cognition, behavior, and mood: Clinical findings and structural-functional synergies with cell membrane phospholipids. *Altern. Med. Rev.* 12, 207–227 (2007).

437. Sublette, M. E., Ellis, S. P., Geant, A. L. & Mann, J. J. Meta-analysis of the effects of eicosapentaenoic acid (EPA) in clinical trials in depression. *J. Clin. Psychiatry* 72, 1577–1584 (2011).

438. Riley, L. W., Raphael, E. & Faerstein, E. Obesity in the United States—dysbiosis from exposure to low-dose antibiotics? *Frontiers in Public Health* 1, 69 (2013).

439. Superbugs Invade American Supermarkets. *Environmental Working Group* (2013). Available at: http://static.ewg.org/reports/2013/meateaters/ewg_meat_and_antibiotics_report2013.pdf. (Accessed: 16th May 2016)

440. Van Boeckel, T. P. et al. Global trends in antimicrobial use in food animals. *Proc. Natl. Acad. Sci. U.S.A.* 112, 5649–5654 (2015).

441. O'Brien, J. J., Campbell, N. & Conaghan, T. Effect of cooking and cold storage on biologically active antibiotic residues in meat. *Journal of Hygiene* 87, 511–523 (1981).

442. Fleming, A. Nobel Lecture. (1945).

443. World Health Organization. Antibiotic Resistance. (2015). Available at: http://www.who.int/mediacentre/factsheets/antibiotic-resistance/en/. (Accessed: 15th April 2016)

444. Markel, H. The Real Story behind Penicillin. *PBS* (2013). Available at: http://www.pbs.org/newshour/rundown/the-real-story-behind-the-worlds-first-antibiotic/. (Accessed: 15th April 2016)

445. Gilbert, N. World's rivers "awash with dangerous levels of antibiotics." *The Guardian* (2019).

446. Casado, J., Brigden, K., Santillo, D. & Johnston, P. Screening of pesticides and veterinary drugs in small streams in the European Union by liquid chromatography high resolution mass spectrometry. *Sci. Total Environ.* 670, 1204–1225 (2019).

447. Review on Antimicrobial Resistance. *Tackling Drug-Resistant Infections Globally: Final Report and Recommendations.* (UK Government, 2016).

448. Średnicka-Tober, D. et al. Composition differences between organic and conventional meat: A systematic literature review and meta-analysis. *Br. J. Nutr.* 115, 994–1011 (2016).

449. Średnicka-Tober, D. et al. Higher PUFA and n-3 PUFA, conjugated linoleic acid, α-tocopherol and iron, but lower iodine and selenium concentrations in organic milk: A systematic literature review and meta- and redundancy analyses. *Br. J. Nutr.* 115, 1043–1060 (2016).

450. Barański, M. et al. Higher antioxidant and lower cadmium concentrations and lower incidence of pesticide residues in organically grown crops: A systematic literature review and meta-analyses. *Br. J. Nutr.* 1–18 (2014).

451. National Center for Complementary and Integrative Health. Antioxidants: In Depth. *National Institutes of Health* (2010). Available at: https://nccih.nih.gov/health/antioxidants/introduction.htm. (Accessed: 19th May 2016)

452. Mosele, J. I., Macià, A. & Motilva, M.-J. Metabolic and microbial modulation of the large intestine ecosystem by non-absorbed diet phenolic compounds: A review. *Molecules* 20, 17429–17468 (2015).

453. Reganold, J. P. et al. Fruit and soil quality of organic and conventional strawberry agroecosystems. *PLoS One* 5, e12346 (2010).

454. Wassermann, B., Müller, H. & Berg, G. An apple a day: Which bacteria do we eat with organic and conventional apples? *Front. Microbiol.* 10, 1629 (2019).

455. Smith-Spangler, C. et al. Are organic foods safer or healthier than conventional alternatives? A systematic review. *Ann. Intern. Med.* 157, 348–366 (2012).

456. Benbrook, C. Initial reflections on the Annals of Internal Medicine paper "Are Organic Foods Safer and Healthier Than Conventional Alternatives? A Systematic Review." *Annals of Internal Medicine* (2012).

457. Dean, A. Stanford-Cargill Partnership Strengthens to Address Food Security. (2011). Available at: https://fse.fsi.stanford.edu/news/stanfordcargill_partnership_strengthens_to_ address_food_security_issues_20111127. (Accessed: 13th November 2019)

458. Organic Food Debunker Was Tobacco Institute Researcher in 1976. Available at: http:// www.thepeoplesvoice.org/TPV3/Voices.php/2012/09/06/organic-food-debunker-was-tobacco-instit-1976. (Accessed: 17th May 2016)

459. Holzman, D. C. Organic food conclusions don't tell the whole story. *Environ. Health Perspect.* 120, A458 (2012).

460. Whyatt, R. M. & Barr, D. B. Measurement of organophosphate metabolites in postpartum meconium as a potential biomarker of prenatal exposure: A validation study. *Environ. Health Perspect.* 109, 417–420 (2001).

461. Schreinemachers, D. M. Birth malformations and other adverse perinatal outcomes in four U.S. wheat-producing states. *Environ. Health Perspect.* 111, 1259–1264 (2003).

462. Arbuckle, T. E., Lin, Z. & Mery, L. S. An exploratory analysis of the effect of pesticide exposure on the risk of spontaneous abortion in an Ontario farm population. *Environ. Health Perspect.* 109, 851–857 (2001).

463. Garry, V. F. et al. Birth defects, season of conception, and sex of children born to pesticide applicators living in the Red River Valley of Minnesota, USA. *Environ. Health Perspect.* 110 Suppl 3, 441–449 (2002).

464. Marquez, E. C. & Schafer, K. S. *Kids on the Frontline—How Pesticides Are Undermining the Health of Rural Children.* (Pesticide Action Network North America, 2016).

465. Rauh, V. et al. Seven-year neurodevelopmental scores and prenatal exposure to chlorpyrifos, a common agricultural pesticide. *Environ. Health Perspect.* 119, 1196–1201 (2011).

466. Bouchard, M. F. et al. Prenatal exposure to organophosphate pesticides and IQ in 7-year-old children. *Environ. Health Perspect.* 119, 1189–1195 (2011).

467. Engel, S. M. et al. Prenatal exposure to organophosphates, paraoxonase 1, and cognitive development in childhood. *Environ. Health Perspect.* 119, 1182–1188 (2011).

468. Mie, A. et al. Human health implications of organic food and organic agriculture: A comprehensive review. *Environ. Health* 16, 111 (2017).

469. Hernández, A. F., Parrón, T. & Alarcón, R. Pesticides and asthma. *Curr. Opin. Allergy Clin. Immunol.* 11, 90–96 (2011).

470. Raanan, R. et al. Decreased lung function in 7-year-old children with early-life organophosphate exposure. *Thorax* 71, 148–153 (2016).

471. Raanan, R. et al. Early-life exposure to organophosphate pesticides and pediatric respiratory symptoms in the CHAMACOS cohort. *Environ. Health Perspect.* 123, 179–185 (2015).

472. Salam, M. T., Li, Y.-F., Langholz, B., Gilliland, F. D. & Children's Health Study. Early-life environmental risk factors for asthma: Findings from the Children's Health Study. *Environ. Health Perspect.* 112, 760–765 (2004).

473. Council on Environmental Health. Pesticide exposure in children. *Pediatrics* 130, e1757–63 (2012).

474. Curl, C. L. et al. Estimating pesticide exposure from dietary intake and organic food choices: The Multi-Ethnic Study of Atherosclerosis (MESA). *Environ. Health Perspect.* 123, 475–483 (2015).

475. Lu, C. et al. Organic diets significantly lower children's dietary exposure to organophosphorus pesticides. *Environ. Health Perspect.* 114, 260–263 (2006).

476. Lu, C., Barr, D. B., Pearson, M. A. & Waller, L. A. Dietary intake and its contribution to longitudinal organophosphorus pesticide exposure in urban/suburban children. *Environ. Health Perspect.* 116, 537–542 (2008).

477. Bradman, A. et al. Effect of organic diet intervention on pesticide exposures in young children living in low-income urban and agricultural communities. *Environ. Health Perspect.* 123, 1086–1093 (2015).

478. Baudry, J. et al. Association of frequency of organic food consumption with cancer risk: Findings from the Nutrinet-Santé prospective cohort study. *JAMA Intern. Med.* 178, 1597–1606 (2018).

479. Shanker, D. Buying Organic Veggies at the Supermarket Is a Waste of Money. *Quartz* (2015). Available at: http://qz.com/488851/buying-organic-veggies-at-the-supermarket-is-basically-a-waste-of-money/. (Accessed: 30th May 2016)

480. Wilcox, C. Mythbusting 101: Organic Farming > Conventional Agriculture. *Scientific American Blog Network* (2011). Available at: http://blogs.scientificamerican.com/science-sushi/httpblogsscientificamericancomscience-sushi20110718mythbusting-101-organic-farming-conventional-agriculture/. (Accessed: 30th May 2016)

481. Oregon State University. *Bacillus thuringiensis. Extension Toxicology Network* (1996). Available at: http://extoxnet.orst.edu/pips/bacillus.htm. (Accessed: 30th May 2016)

482. Entomological Society of America. *Is Bt Safe for Humans to Eat?* (2018).

483. Mark, J. Myths: Busted—Clearing Up the Misunderstandings about Organic Farming. *Scientific American Blog Network* (2011). Available at: http://blogs.scientificamerican.com/guest-blog/myths-busted-clearing-up-the-misunderstandings-about-organic-farming/. (Accessed: 19th May 2016)

484. Greenpeace. Pestizidvergleich: Ist Bio Besser? *Greenpeace* (2007). Available at: https://www.greenpeace.de/themen/landwirtschaft/pestizide/pestizidvergleich-ist-bio-besser. (Accessed: 2016)

485. Badgley, C. et al. Organic agriculture and the global food supply. *Renew. Agric. Food Syst.* 22, 86–108 (2007).

486. Rodale Institute. Farming Systems Trial: Overview. *Rodale Institute* (2015). Available at: http://rodaleinstitute.org/our-work/farming-systems-trial/. (Accessed: 30th May 2016)

487. Russell, K. & Hakim, D. Broken Promises of Genetically Modified Crops. *The New York Times* (2016).

488. United Nations Human Rights Council. *Eco-Farming Can Double Food Production in 10 Years, Says New UN Report.* (United Nations, 2011).

489. Carrington, D. UN experts denounce "myth" pesticides are necessary to feed the world. *The Guardian* (2017).

490. Carrington, D. Plummeting insect numbers "threaten collapse of nature." *The Guardian* (2019).

491. Watts, J. We have 12 years to limit climate change catastrophe, warns UN. *The Guardian* (2018).

492. Wallace-Wells, D. *The Uninhabitable Earth: Life after Warming.* (Tim Duggan Books, 2019).

493. Carrington, D. Buy organic food to help curb global insect collapse, say scientists. *The Guardian* (2019).

494. Hickel, J. Our best shot at cooling the planet might be right under our feet. *The Guardian* (2016).

495. Harvey, F. Switching to organic farming could cut greenhouse gas emissions, study shows. *The Guardian* (2017).

496. EWG Dirty Dozen. *Environmental Working Group* (2016). Available at: https://www.ewg.org/foodnews/dirty_dozen_list.php.

497. Removing Pesticides from Fruits and Vegetables. *Centre for Science and Environment* Available at: http://www.cseindia.org/node/2681. (Accessed: 20th May 2016)

498. EWG Clean Fifteen. *Environmental Working Group* (2016). Available at: https://www.ewg.org/foodnews/clean_fifteen_list.php.

499. Creasy, R. & Wilkinson Barash, C. Edible Landscaping: Grow $700 of Food in 100 Square Feet! *Mother Earth News* (2010). Available at: http://www.motherearthnews.com/organic-gardening/edible-landscaping-zmaz09djzraw.aspx?PageId=1. (Accessed: 20th May 2016)

500. Lowry, C. A. et al. Identification of an immune-responsive mesolimbocortical serotonergic system: Potential role in regulation of emotional behavior. *Neuroscience* 146, 756–772 (2007).

501. Glausiuz, J. Is Dirt the New Prozac? *Discover Magazine* (2007). Available at: http://discovermagazine.com/2007/jul/raw-data-is-dirt-the-new-prozac. (Accessed: 20th May 2016)

502. Can Bacteria Make You Smarter? *ScienceDaily* (2010). Available at: https://www.sciencedaily.com/releases/2010/05/100524143416.htm. (Accessed: 20th May 2016)

503. Cisternas, M. G. et al. A comprehensive study of the direct and indirect costs of adult asthma. *Journal of Allergy and Clinical Immunology* 111, 1212–1218 (2003).

504. Cleaning Supplies and Your Health. *Environmental Working Group* (2016). Available at: http://www.ewg.org/guides/cleaners/content/cleaners_and_health. (Accessed: 12th April 2016)

505. Zock, J.-P. et al. The use of household cleaning sprays and adult asthma: An international longitudinal study. *Am. J. Respir. Crit. Care Med.* 176, 735–741 (2007).

506. Sherriff, A., Farrow, A., Golding, J. & Henderson, J. Frequent use of chemical household products is associated with persistent wheezing in pre-school age children. *Thorax* 60, 45–49 (2005).

507. Svanes, Ø. et al. Cleaning at home and at work in relation to lung function decline and airway obstruction. *Am. J. Respir. Crit. Care Med.* 197, 1157–1163 (2018).

508. Gascon, M. et al. Prenatal exposure to bisphenol A and phthalates and childhood respiratory tract infections and allergy. *J. Allergy Clin. Immunol.* 135, 370–378 (2015).

509. Phthalates. *Campaign for Safe Cosmetics* (2016). Available at: http://www.safecosmetics.org/get-the-facts/chemicals-of-concern/phthalates/. (Accessed: 13th April 2016)

510. Parabens. *Campaign for Safe Cosmetics* (2016). Available at: http://www.safecosmetics.org/get-the-facts/chemicals-of-concern/parabens/. (Accessed: 13th April 2016)

511. Caress, S. M. & Steinemann, A. C. Prevalence of fragrance sensitivity in the American population. *J. Environ. Health* 71, 46–50 (2009).

512. Pasch, E., Voltmer, L., Gemmell, S., Walter, J. & Walton, K. L. W. Effects of triclosan on the normal intestinal microbiota and on susceptibility to experimental murine colitis. *The FASEB Journal* 23, 977.10–977.10 (2009).

513. Bertelsen, R. J. et al. Triclosan exposure and allergic sensitization in Norwegian children. *Allergy* 68, 84–91 (2013).

514. Savage, J. H., Matsui, E. C., Wood, R. A. & Keet, C. A. Urinary levels of triclosan and parabens are associated with aeroallergen and food sensitization. *J. Allergy Clin. Immunol.* 130, 453–60.e7 (2012).

515. Calafat, A. M., Ye, X., Wong, L.-Y., Reidy, J. A. & Needham, L. L. Urinary concentrations of triclosan in the U.S. population: 2003–2004. *Environ. Health Perspect.* 116, 303–307 (2008).

516. Dayan, A. D. Risk assessment of triclosan [Irgasan®] in human breast milk. *Food Chem. Toxicol.* 45, 125–129 (2007).

517. Allmyr, M., Adolfsson-Erici, M., McLachlan, M. S. & Sandborgh-Englund, G. Triclosan in plasma and milk from Swedish nursing mothers and their exposure via personal care products. *Sci. Total Environ.* 372, 87–93 (2006).

518. Aiello, A. E., Larson, E. L. & Levy, S. B. Consumer antibacterial soaps: Effective or just risky? *Clin. Infect. Dis.* 45 Suppl 2, S137–47 (2007).

519. Yazdankhah, S. P. et al. Triclosan and antimicrobial resistance in bacteria: An overview. *Microb. Drug Resist.* 12, 83–90 (2006).

520. Sreevidya, V. S., Lenz, K. A., Svoboda, K. R. & Ma, H. Benzalkonium chloride, benzethonium chloride, and chloroxylenol—three replacement antimicrobials are more toxic than triclosan and triclocarban in two model organisms. *Environ. Pollut.* 235, 814–824 (2018).

521. Herdt-Losavio, M. L. et al. Maternal occupation and the risk of birth defects: An overview from the National Birth Defects Prevention Study. *Occup. Environ. Med.* 67, 58–66 (2010).

522. Chemicals of Concern. *Campaign for Safe Cosmetics* (2019). Available at: http://www. safecosmetics.org/get-the-facts/chem-of-concern/.

523. Formaldehyde. *Environmental Protection Agency* (2000). Available at: https://www3.epa. gov/airtoxics/hlthef/formalde.html. (Accessed: 13th April 2016)

524. Formaldehyde and Cancer Risk. *National Cancer Institute* (2011). Available at: http://www. cancer.gov/about-cancer/causes-prevention/risk/substances/formaldehyde/formaldehyde-fact-sheet. (Accessed: 13th April 2016)

525. Formaldehyde and Formaldehyde-Releasing Preservatives. *Campaign for Safe Cosmetics* (2016). Available at: http://www.safecosmetics.org/get-the-facts/chemicals-of-concern/ formaldehyde/. (Accessed: 13th April 2016)

526. US Laws. *Campaign for Safe Cosmetics* (2016). Available at: http://www.safecosmetics.org/ get-the-facts/regulations/us-laws/. (Accessed: 18th April 2016)

527. Myths on Cosmetics Safety. *Environmental Working Group* (2016). Available at: http://www. ewg.org/skindeep/myths-on-cosmetics-safety/. (Accessed: 15th April 2016)

528. Health Canada. Cosmetic Ingredient Hotlist. (2015). Available at: http://www.hc-sc.gc.ca/ cps-spc/cosmet-person/hot-list-critique/hotlist-liste-eng.php. (Accessed: 18th April 2016)

529. International Laws. *Campaign for Safe Cosmetics* (2016). Available at: http://www. safecosmetics.org/get-the-facts/regulations/international-laws/. (Accessed: 18th April 2016)

530. Environmental Defence. Heavy Metal Hazard: The Health Risks of Hidden Heavy Metals in Face Makeup. *Environmental Defence* (2011). Available at: http://environmentaldefence. ca/report/report-heavy-metal-hazard-the-health-risks-of-hidden-heavy-metals-in-face-makeup/. (Accessed: 7th June 2016)

531. Methylisothiazolinone and Methylchloroisothiazolinone. *Campaign for Safe Cosmetics* (2016). Available at: http://www.safecosmetics.org/get-the-facts/chemicals-of-concern/ methylisothiazolinone/. (Accessed: 15th April 2016)

532. Castanedo-Tardana, M. P. & Zug, K. A. Methylisothiazolinone. *Dermatitis* 24, 2–6 (2013).

533. Cahill, J. L., Toholka, R. W. & Nixon, R. L. Methylisothiazolinone in baby wipes: A rising star among causes of contact dermatitis. *Med. J. Aust.* 200, 208 (2014).

534. He, K., Huang, J., Lagenaur, C. F. & Aizenman, E. Methylisothiazolinone, a neurotoxic biocide, disrupts the association of SRC family tyrosine kinases with focal adhesion kinase in developing cortical neurons. *J. Pharmacol. Exp. Ther.* 317, 1320–1329 (2006).

535. Anderson, R. C. & Anderson, J. H. Acute respiratory effects of diaper emissions. *Arch. Environ. Health* 54, 353–358 (1999).

536. Alberta, L., Sweeney, S. M. & Wiss, K. Diaper dye dermatitis. *Pediatrics* 116, e450–2 (2005).

537. DeVito, M. J. & Schecter, A. Exposure assessment to dioxins from the use of tampons and diapers. *Environ. Health Perspect.* 110, 23–28 (2002).

538. Spurrier, J. What Is Inside Those Disposable Diapers? *BabyGearLab.com* (2014). Available at: http://www.babygearlab.com/a/11113/What-Is-Inside-Those-Disposable-Diapers. (Accessed: 21st April 2016)

539. World Health Organization. Dioxins and Their Effects on Human Health. (2014). Available at: http://www.who.int/mediacentre/factsheets/fs225/en/. (Accessed: 21st April 2016)

540. The Clorox Company. Green Works® Naturally Derived All-Purpose Cleaner. (2016). Available at: https://www.thecloroxcompany.com/products/ingredients-inside/en-us/greenworks/greenworksnaturallyderivedallpurposecleaner/. (Accessed: 19th April 2016)

541. Synthetic Musks. *Campaign for Safe Cosmetics* (2016). Available at: http://www.safecosmetics.org/get-the-facts/chemicals-of-concern/synthetic-musks/. (Accessed: 19th April 2016)

542. The Clorox Company. Fragrances—Ingredients Inside. (2016). Available at: https://www.thecloroxcompany.com/products/ingredients-inside/fragrances/en-us/. (Accessed: 19th April 2016)

543. Environmental Working Group. Green Works Naturally Derived All-Purpose Cleaner, Original—Cleaner Rating. *EWG's Guide to Healthy Cleaning* (2016). Available at: http://www.ewg.org/guides/cleaners/568-GreenWorksnaturallyderivedallpurposecleaneroriginal?formulation=6792. (Accessed: 19th April 2016)

544. Honaker, B. Huggies Class Action Says Snug & Dry Diapers Cause Rash. *Top Class Actions* (2018). Available at: https://topclassactions.com/lawsuit-settlements/lawsuit-news/855498-huggies-class-action-says-snug-dry-diapers-cause-rash/. (Accessed: 4th June 2019)

545. Huggies Natural Baby Wipes. *Truth in Advertising* (2018). Available at: https://www.truthinadvertising.org/huggies-natural-baby-wipes/. (Accessed: 4th June 2019)

546. Environmental Working Group. Huggies Natural Care Baby Wipes, Fragrance Free. *Skin Deep® Cosmetics Database* (2013). Available at: http://www.ewg.org/skindeep/product/1417/Huggies_Natural_Care_Baby_Wipes,_Fragrance_Free/. (Accessed: 21st April 2016)

547. Unacceptable Ingredients for Cleaning Products. *Whole Foods Market* (2014). Available at: http://www.wholefoodsmarket.com/mission-values/environmental-stewardship/eco-scale/unacceptable-ingredients. (Accessed: 20th April 2016)

548. Premium Body Care Standards. *Whole Foods Market* (2015). Available at: http://www.wholefoodsmarket.com/about-our-products/premium-body-care-standards. (Accessed: 20th April 2016)

549. Amorim, J. L. et al. Anti-inflammatory properties and chemical characterization of the essential oils of four citrus species. *PLoS One* 11, e0153643 (2016).

550. Sarmento-Neto, J. F., do Nascimento, L. G., Felipe, C. F. B. & de Sousa, D. P. Analgesic potential of essential oils. *Molecules* 21, E20 (2015).

551. Cho, K. S. et al. Terpenes from forests and human health. *Toxicol. Res.* 33, 97–106 (2017).

552. Dagli, N., Dagli, R., Mahmoud, R. S. & Baroudi, K. Essential oils, their therapeutic properties, and implication in dentistry: A review. *J. Int. Soc. Prev. Community Dent.* 5, 335–340 (2015).

553. Lillehei, A. S. & Halcon, L. L. A systematic review of the effect of inhaled essential oils on sleep. *J. Altern. Complement. Med.* 20, 441–451 (2014).

554. Wang, Z.-J. & Heinbockel, T. Essential oils and their constituents targeting the GABAergic system and sodium channels as treatment of neurological diseases. *Molecules* 23 (2018).

555. Dosoky, N. S. & Setzer, W. N. Biological activities and safety of citrus spp. essential oils. *Int. J. Mol. Sci.* 19 (2018).

556. Soloway, R. A. G. Essential Oils: Poisonous When Misused. *National Capital Poison Center* (2014). Available at: https://poison.org/articles/2014%20jun/essential%20oils. (Accessed: 11th November 2019)

557. Irritation and Allergic Reactions to Essential Oils. *Tisserand Institute* (2019). Available at: https://tisserandinstitute.org/safety/irritation-allergic-reactions/. (Accessed: 11th November 2019)

558. How to Use Essential Oils Safely. *Tisserand Institute* (2019). Available at: https://tisserandinstitute.org/safety/safety-guidelines/. (Accessed: 11th November 2019)

559. Matura, M. et al. Selected oxidized fragrance terpenes are common contact allergens. *Contact Dermatitis* 52, 320–328 (2005).

560. de Groot, A. C. & Schmidt, E. Essential oils, part IV: Contact allergy. *Dermatitis* 27, 170–175 (2016).

561. Tisserand, R. Lemon on the Rocks: Keep Your Essential Oils Cool. *Robert Tisserand* (2013). Available at: https://roberttisserand.com/2013/07/lemon-on-the-rockskeep-your-essential-oils-cool/. (Accessed: 11th November 2019)

562. Singh, G. & Archana, G. Unraveling the mystery of vernix caseosa. *Indian Journal of Dermatology* 53, 54–60 (2008).

563. Lieberman, S., Enig, M. G. & Preuss, P. H. G. A review of monolaurin and lauric acid: Natural virucidal and bactericidal agents. *Alternative & Complementary Therapies* 12, 310–314 (2006).

564. Ogbolu, D. O., Oni, A. A., Daini, O. A. & Oloko, A. P. In vitro antimicrobial properties of coconut oil on *Candida* species in Ibadan, Nigeria. *Journal of Medicinal Foods* 10, 384–387 (2007).

565. Verallo-Rowell, V. M., Dillague, K. M. & Syah-Tjundawan, B. S. Novel antibacterial and emollient effects of coconut and virgin olive oils in adult atopic dermatitis. *Dermatitis* 19, 308–315 (2008).

566. Glenza, J. Why does it cost $32,093 just to give birth in America? *The Guardian* (2018).

567. McDermott, S. The real cost of giving birth: "I had to pay $40 to hold my newborn baby." *BBC News* (2016). Available at: http://www.bbc.com/news/blogs-trending-37555048. (Accessed: 11th September 2017)

568. Betrán, A. P. et al. The increasing trend in caesarean section rates: Global, regional and national estimates: 1990–2014. *PLoS One* 11, e0148343 (2016).

569. Bager, P., Wohlfahrt, J. & Westergaard, T. Caesarean delivery and risk of atopy and allergic disease: Meta-analyses. *Clin. Exp. Allergy* 38, 634–642 (2008).

570. Thavagnanam, S., Fleming, J., Bromley, A., Shields, M. D. & Cardwell, C. R. A meta-analysis of the association between caesarean section and childhood asthma. *Clinical & Experimental Allergy* 38, 629–633 (2008).

571. O'Neill, S. M. et al. Birth by caesarean section and the risk of adult psychosis: A population-based cohort study. *Schizophr. Bull.* 42, 633–641 (2016).

572. Cardwell, C. R. et al. Caesarean section is associated with an increased risk of childhood-onset type 1 diabetes mellitus: A meta-analysis of observational studies. *Diabetologia* 51, 726–735 (2008).

573. Sevelsted, A., Stokholm, J., Bønnelykke, K. & Bisgaard, H. Cesarean section and chronic immune disorders. *Pediatrics* eds.2014-0596-(2014).

574. Cho, C. E. & Norman, M. Cesarean section and development of the immune system in the offspring. *Am. J. Obstet. Gynecol.* 208, 249–254 (2013).

575. Kapoor, A., Dunn, E., Kostaki, A., Andrews, M. H. & Matthews, S. G. Fetal programming of hypothalamo-pituitary-adrenal function: Prenatal stress and glucocorticoids. *J. Physiol.* 572, 31–44 (2006).

576. Bråbäck, L., Lowe, A. & Hjern, A. Elective cesarean section and childhood asthma. *Am. J. Obstet. Gynecol.* 209, 496 (2013).

577. Shin, H. et al. The first microbial environment of infants born by C-section: The operating room microbes. *Microbiome* 3, 59 (2015).

578. Mueller, N. T., Bakacs, E., Combellick, J., Grigoryan, Z. & Dominguez-Bello, M. G. The infant microbiome development: Mom matters. *Trends Mol. Med.* 21, 109–117 (2014).

579. Grönlund, M. M., Lehtonen, O. P., Eerola, E. & Kero, P. Fecal microflora in healthy infants born by different methods of delivery: Permanent changes in intestinal flora after cesarean delivery. *J. Pediatr. Gastroenterol. Nutr.* 28, 19–25 (1999).

580. Salminen, S., Gibson, G. R., McCartney, A. L. & Isolauri, E. Influence of mode of delivery on gut microbiota composition in seven year old children. *Gut* 53, 1388–1389 (2004).

581. Andrews, W. W., Hauth, J. C., Cliver, S. P., Savage, K. & Goldenberg, R. L. Randomized clinical trial of extended spectrum antibiotic prophylaxis with coverage for *Ureaplasma urealyticum* to reduce post-cesarean delivery endometritis. *Obstet. Gynecol.* 101, 1183–1189 (2003).

582. Ledger, W. J. & Blaser, M. J. Are we using too many antibiotics during pregnancy? *BJOG* 120, 1450–1452 (2013).

583. Dominguez-Bello, M. G. et al. Partial restoration of the microbiota of cesarean-born infants via vaginal microbial transfer. *Nat. Med.* 22, 250–253 (2016).

584. Clemente, J. C. & Dominguez-Bello, M. G. Safety of vaginal microbial transfer in infants delivered by caesarean, and expected health outcomes. *BMJ* 352, i1707 (2016).

585. Stinson, L. F., Payne, M. S. & Keelan, J. A. A critical review of the bacterial baptism hypothesis and the impact of cesarean delivery on the infant microbiome. *Front. Med.* 5, 135 (2018).

586. Hodnett, E. D., Gates, S., Hofmeyr, G. J. & Sakala, C. Continuous support for women during childbirth. *Cochrane Database Syst. Rev.* 7, CD003766 (2013).

587. Steel, A. et al. The value of care provided by student doulas: An examination of the perceptions of women in their care. *J. Perinat. Educ.* 22, 39–48 (2013).

588. Larsson, P. G., Platz-Christensen, J. J., Bergman, B. & Wallstersson, G. Advantage or disadvantage of episiotomy compared with spontaneous perineal laceration. *Gynecol. Obstet. Invest.* 31, 213–216 (1991).

589. Andersson, O., Hellström-Westas, L., Andersson, D. & Domellöf, M. Effect of delayed versus early umbilical cord clamping on neonatal outcomes and iron status at 4 months: A randomised controlled trial. *BMJ* 343, d7157 (2011).

590. Andersson, O. et al. Effect of delayed cord clamping on neurodevelopment at 4 years of age. *JAMA Pediatr.* 169, 631 (2015).

591. Zielinski, R., Ackerson, K. & Kane Low, L. Planned home birth: Benefits, risks, and opportunities. *Int. J. Women's Health* 7, 361–377 (2015).

592. Royal College of Obstetricians and Gynaecologists & Royal College of Midwives. Home Births—Joint Statement. (2007).

593. Lawrence, R. M. & Lawrence, R. A. Breastfeeding: More than just good nutrition. *Pediatr. Rev.* 32, 267–280 (2011).

594. World Health Organization. Exclusive Breastfeeding. *WHO* (2017). Available at: http://www.who.int/nutrition/topics/exclusive_breastfeeding/en/. (Accessed: 22nd November 2017)

595. Sample, I. Baby boys and girls receive different nutrients in breast milk. *The Guardian* (2014).

596. Geddes, L. Evening breast milk means a good sleep. *New Scientist* (2009).

597. Sánchez, C. L. et al. The possible role of human milk nucleotides as sleep inducers. *Nutr. Neurosci.* 12, 2–8 (2009).

598. Kimata, H. Laughter elevates the levels of breast-milk melatonin. *J. Psychosom. Res.* 62, 699–702 (2007).

599. Al-Shehri, S. S. et al. Breastmilk-saliva interactions boost innate immunity by regulating the oral microbiome in early infancy. *PLoS One* 10, e0135047 (2015).

600. Ghosh, M. K., Nguyen, V., Muller, H. K. & Walker, A. M. Maternal milk T cells drive development of transgenerational Th1 immunity in offspring thymus. *J. Immunol.* **197**, 2290–2296 (2016).

601. University of California–Riverside. Vaccinating babies without vaccinating babies: A baby makes copies of maternal immune cells it acquires through mother's milk. *Science Daily* (2016).

602. Medical College of Georgia at Augusta University. SWAT team of immune cells found in mother's milk. *Science Daily* (2018).

603. Baban, B., Malik, A., Bhatia, J. & Yu, J. C. Presence and profile of innate lymphoid cells in human breast milk. *JAMA Pediatr.* **172**, 594–596 (2018).

604. Artis, D. & Spits, H. The biology of innate lymphoid cells. *Nature* **517**, 293–301 (2015).

605. Butler, J. E. Immunologic aspects of breast feeding, antiinfectious activity of breast milk. *Semin. Perinatol.* **3**, 255–270 (1979).

606. Chirico, G., Marzollo, R., Cortinovis, S., Fonte, C. & Gasparoni, A. Antiinfective properties of human milk. *The Journal of Nutrition* **138**, 1801S–1806S (2008).

607. Chen, A. & Rogan, W. J. Breastfeeding and the risk of postneonatal death in the United States. *Pediatrics* **113**, e435–9 (2004).

608. Duijts, L., Jaddoe, V. W. V., Hofman, A. & Moll, H. A. Prolonged and exclusive breastfeeding reduces the risk of infectious diseases in infancy. *Pediatrics* **126**, e18–25 (2010).

609. Duijts, L., Ramadhani, M. K. & Moll, H. A. Breastfeeding protects against infectious diseases during infancy in industrialized countries. A systematic review. *Matern. Child Nutr.* **5**, 199–210 (2009).

610. NEOVITA Study Group. Timing of initiation, patterns of breastfeeding, and infant survival: Prospective analysis of pooled data from three randomised trials. *Lancet Global Health* **4**, e266–75 (2016).

611. Hörnell, A., Lagström, H., Lande, B. & Thorsdottir, I. Breastfeeding, introduction of other foods and effects on health: A systematic literature review for the 5th Nordic Nutrition Recommendations. *Food Nutr. Res.* **57** (2013).

612. Pacheco, A. R., Barile, D., Underwood, M. A. & Mills, D. A. The impact of the milk glycobiome on the neonate gut microbiota. *Annu. Rev. Anim. Biosci.* **3**, 419–445 (2015).

613. Klopp, A. et al. Modes of infant feeding and the risk of childhood asthma: A prospective birth cohort study. *J. Pediatr.* **190**, 192–199.e2 (2017).

614. Ehlayel, M. S. & Bener, A. Duration of breast-feeding and the risk of childhood allergic diseases in a developing country. *Allergy Asthma Proc.* **29**, 386–391 (2008).

615. Bener, A., Ehlayel, M. S., Alsowaidi, S. & Sabbah, A. Role of breast feeding in primary prevention of asthma and allergic diseases in a traditional society. *Eur. Ann. Allergy Clin. Immunol.* **39**, 337–343 (2007).

616. Snijders, B. E. P. et al. Breast-feeding duration and infant atopic manifestations, by maternal allergic status, in the first 2 years of life (KOALA study). *J. Pediatr.* 151, 347–51, 351. e1–2 (2007).

617. Gdalevich, M., Mimouni, D. & Mimouni, M. Breast-feeding and the risk of bronchial asthma in childhood: A systematic review with meta-analysis of prospective studies. *J. Pediatr.* 139, 261–266 (2001).

618. Gdalevich, M., Mimouni, D., David, M. & Mimouni, M. Breast-feeding and the onset of atopic dermatitis in childhood: A systematic review and meta-analysis of prospective studies. *J. Am. Acad. Dermatol.* 45, 520–527 (2001).

619. Oddy, W. H. et al. Association between breast feeding and asthma in 6 year old children: Findings of a prospective birth cohort study. *BMJ* 319, 815–819 (1999).

620. Saarinen, U. M. & Kajosaari, M. Breastfeeding as prophylaxis against atopic disease: Prospective follow-up study until 17 years old. *Lancet* 346, 1065–1069 (1995).

621. Dell, S. & To, T. Breastfeeding and asthma in young children: Findings from a population-based study. *Arch. Pediatr. Adolesc. Med.* 155, 1261–1265 (2001).

622. Rothenbacher, D., Weyermann, M., Beermann, C. & Brenner, H. Breastfeeding, soluble CD14 concentration in breast milk and risk of atopic dermatitis and asthma in early childhood: Birth cohort study. *Clin. Exp. Allergy* 35, 1014–1021 (2005).

623. Klement, E., Cohen, R. V., Boxman, J., Joseph, A. & Reif, S. Breastfeeding and risk of inflammatory bowel disease: A systematic review with meta-analysis. *Am. J. Clin. Nutr.* 80, 1342–1352 (2004).

624. Ley, R. E. Obesity and the human microbiome. *Curr. Opin. Gastroenterol.* 26, 5–11 (2010).

625. Woo, J. G. & Martin, L. J. Does breastfeeding protect against childhood obesity? Moving beyond observational evidence. *Curr. Obes. Rep.* 4, 207–216 (2015).

626. Amitay, E. L. & Keinan-Boker, L. Breastfeeding and childhood leukemia incidence: A meta-analysis and systematic review. *JAMA Pediatr.* 169, e151025 (2015).

627. Martin, R. M., Gunnell, D., Owen, C. G. & Smith, G. D. Breast-feeding and childhood cancer: A systematic review with metaanalysis. *Int. J. Cancer* 117, 1020–1031 (2005).

628. Knapton, S. Breast milk chemical dissolves tumours so cancer patients can pass them in urine, trial shows. *The Daily Telegraph* (2019).

629. Victora, C. G. et al. Association between breastfeeding and intelligence, educational attainment, and income at 30 years of age: A prospective birth cohort study from Brazil. *The Lancet Global Health* 3, e199–e205 (2015).

630. Skugarevsky, O. et al. Effects of promoting longer-term and exclusive breastfeeding on childhood eating attitudes: A cluster-randomized trial. *Int. J. Epidemiol.* 43, 1263–1271 (2014).

631. Mezzacappa, E. S. Breastfeeding and maternal stress response and health. *Nutr. Rev.* 62, 261–268 (2004).

632. Gribble, K. D. Mental health, attachment and breastfeeding: Implications for adopted children and their mothers. *Int. Breastfeed. J.* 1, 5 (2006).

633. Groer, M. W. & Davis, M. W. Cytokines, infections, stress, and dysphoric moods in breastfeeders and formula feeders. *J. Obstet. Gynecol. Neonatal Nurs.* 35, 599–607 (2006).

634. Weaver, J. M., Schofield, T. J. & Papp, L. M. Breastfeeding duration predicts greater maternal sensitivity over the next decade. *Dev. Psychol.* (2017). doi:10.1037/dev0000425

635. Doan, T., Gay, C. L., Kennedy, H. P., Newman, J. & Lee, K. A. Nighttime breastfeeding behavior is associated with more nocturnal sleep among first-time mothers at one month postpartum. *J. Clin. Sleep Med.* 10, 313–319 (2014).

636. Hansen, K. Breastfeeding: A smart investment in people and in economies. *Lancet* 387, 416 (2016).

637. Kaplan, D. L. & Graff, K. M. Marketing breastfeeding—reversing corporate influence on infant feeding practices. *J. Urban Health* 85, 486–504 (2008).

638. Hill, M. How the billion pound formula industry hijacked breastfeeding. *The Daily Telegraph* (2015).

639. Howard, C. et al. Office prenatal formula advertising and its effect on breast-feeding patterns. *Obstet. Gynecol.* 95, 296–303 (2000).

640. Rosenberg, K. D., Eastham, C. A., Kasehagen, L. J. & Sandoval, A. P. Marketing infant formula through hospitals: The impact of commercial hospital discharge packs on breastfeeding. *Am. J. Public Health* 98, 290–295 (2008).

641. Ellis-Petersen, H. How formula milk firms target mothers who can least afford it. *The Guardian* (2018).

642. Messner, A. H., Lalakea, M. L., Aby, J., Macmahon, J. & Bair, E. Ankyloglossia: Incidence and associated feeding difficulties. *Arch. Otolaryngol. Head. Neck Surg.* 126, 36–39 (2000).

643. O'Shea, J. E. et al. Frenotomy for tongue-tie in newborn infants. *Cochrane Database Syst. Rev.* 3, CD011065 (2017).

644. Kim, J. & Unger, S. Human milk banking. *Paediatr. Child Health* 15, 595–602 (2010).

645. Jang, H. L. et al. The experience of human milk banking for 8 years: Korean perspective. *J. Korean Med. Sci.* 31, 1775–1783 (2016).

646. Colombo, J., Jill Shaddy, D., Kerling, E. H., Gustafson, K. M. & Carlson, S. E. Docosahexaenoic acid (DHA) and arachidonic acid (ARA) balance in developmental outcomes. *Prostaglandins Leukot. Essent. Fatty Acids* 121, 52–56 (2017).

647. de Moura, P. N. & Rosário Filho, N. A. The use of prebiotics during the first year of life for atopy prevention and treatment. *Immun. Inflamm. Dis.* 1, 63–69 (2013).

648. Osborn, D. A. & Sinn, J. Prebiotics in infants for prevention of allergy. *The Cochrane Library* (2013).

649. Cuello-Garcia, C. et al. Prebiotics for the prevention of allergies: A systematic review and meta-analysis of randomized controlled trials. *Clin. Exp. Allergy* 47, 1468–1477 (2017).

650. Brosseau, C. et al. Prebiotics: Mechanisms and preventive effects in allergy. *Nutrients* 11 (2019).

651. Sohn, K. & Underwood, M. A. Prenatal and postnatal administration of prebiotics and probiotics. *Semin. Fetal Neonatal Med.* 22, 284–289 (2017).

652. Bertelsen, R. J., Jensen, E. T. & Ringel-Kulka, T. Use of probiotics and prebiotics in infant feeding. *Best Pract. Res. Clin. Gastroenterol.* 30, 39–48 (2016).

653. Fleischer, D. M., Spergel, J. M., Assa'ad, A. H. & Pongracic, J. A. Primary prevention of allergic disease through nutritional interventions. *J. Allergy Clin. Immunol. Pract.* 1, 29–36 (2013).

654. Szajewska, H. & Horvath, A. A partially hydrolyzed 100% whey formula and the risk of eczema and any allergy: An updated meta-analysis. *World Allergy Organ. J.* 10, 27 (2017).

655. Bhatia, J., Greer, F. & American Academy of Pediatrics Committee on Nutrition. Use of soy protein-based formulas in infant feeding. *Pediatrics* 121, 1062–1068 (2008).

656. Osborn, D. A. & Sinn, J. Soy formula for prevention of allergy and food intolerance in infants. *Cochrane Database Syst. Rev.* CD003741 (2006).

657. National Institutes of Health Staff. Soy Infant Formula. *National Institute of Environmental Health Services* (2017). Available at: https://www.niehs.nih.gov/health/topics/agents/sya-soy-formula/index.cfm. (Accessed: 12th February 2018)

658. Jefferson, W. N., Patisaul, H. B. & Williams, C. J. Reproductive consequences of developmental phytoestrogen exposure. *Reproduction* 143, 247–260 (2012).

659. Strom, B. L. et al. Exposure to soy-based formula in infancy and endocrinological and reproductive outcomes in young adulthood. *JAMA* 286, 807–814 (2001).

660. Goldman, L. R., Newbold, R. & Swan, S. H. Exposure to soy-based formula in infancy. *JAMA* 286, 2402–2403 (2001).

661. Koplin, J. J. & Allen, K. J. Optimal timing for solids introduction—why are the guidelines always changing? *Clin. Exp. Allergy* 43, 826–834 (2013).

662. Sansotta, N. et al. Timing of introduction of solid food and risk of allergic disease development: Understanding the evidence. *Allergol. Immunopathol.* 41, 337–345 (2013).

663. Grimshaw, K. E. C. et al. Introduction of complementary foods and the relationship to food allergy. *Pediatrics* 132, e1529–38 (2013).

664. University of Southampton. Introducing solid foods while continuing to breast feed could prevent child allergies. *Science Daily* (2013).

665. Roberts, M. Baby weaning foods found "lacking." *BBC* (2013).

666. Barone, J. E. Comparing apples and oranges: A randomised prospective study. *BMJ* 321, 1569–1570 (2000).

INDEX

A

absolute risk, 12–13, 225–228

acetate, 35–36, 46–47, 80–81

adrenal glands, 37, 183–184

air fresheners, 162–163

ALA (alpha-linolenic acid), 94, 143

alcohol consumption, 45

Alexander, Albert, 148–149

algae, 94

allergies and atopic diseases, 19–28. *See also* asthma; eczema

    allergic rhinitis, 23–24, 52, 140, 152, 183

    antibiotic use and, 218–219. *See also* antibiotics

    asthma. *See* asthma

    biggest effect on risk for, 233–243

    breastfeeding and, 201. *See also* breastfeeding

    causes of, 24–28

    C-sections and, 183

    dairy consumption and, 102

    development of, 24–27

    eczema. *See* eczema

    fish oil and, 142. *See also* fish oil; omega-3 fatty acids

    food allergies. *See* food allergies

    infant formulas and, 211–212

    lifestyle choices and, 217–222

    nutrient deficiencies during pregnancy and, 229–231

    probiotics and, 139–141

    supplements and, 121

    symptoms and prevalence of, 23–24

    weaning and, 213–214

    yoghurt, fermented foods and, 81

Alpha1H, 202

alpha-tocopherol (vitamin E), 136–137

American Academy of Pediatrics (AAP), 66, 153, 210

American Contact Dermatitis Society, 167

American Heart Association, 100

anaphylactic shock, 23–24, 139–140

animals

    contact with, 49–50, 221, 242–243

    farming, antibiotics in, 147–149

ankyloglossia (tongue-tie), 206–207

antibacterial products, 163–164

antibiotics, 51–74

    in animal farming, 147–149

    antibiotic resistant bacteria, 52, 70, 148

    for bacterial vaginosis (BV), 56–58

    during breastfeeding, 60–66

    broad-spectrum, 51–52

    for children, 2, 66–69

    C-sections and, 184–185

    for endometritis, 60–61

    for Group B *Streptococcus*, 54–56

    for mastitis, 62–64

    microbiome, threat to, 51–54

    overuse of, 51–54

    penicillin, 148–149

    probiotics and, 66, 69–75

    risk of atopic disease and, 218–219, 233–234

    side effects of, 70

F

farmers' markets, 157
farming, antibiotics and, 147–149
fat cells, 112
fats and fatty acids, 85–105
    artificial and trans fats, 104–105
    in breast milk, 197
    cheat sheet for, 87
    fish as source of omega-3s, 96–99
    function of, 85–86
    good, 118
    in infant formula, 211
    monounsaturated fats (MUFA), 88–91
    omega-3 fatty acids. *See* omega-3 fatty acids
    omega-6 fatty acids, 86–87, 90–96
    polyunsaturated fats (PUFA), 86–87, 90–96
    saturated fats, 99–104
    short-chain fatty acids (SCFAs), 35–36, 46–47, 80–81
    sugar and, 110
feeding good bacteria, 77–83. *See also* good bacteria
    dietary fibre, 77–81
    yoghurt and fermented foods, 81–83
fermented foods, 81–83, 102, 142, 220. *See also* yoghurt
fertility problems, 125, 162, 213
fibre
    added fibre, 79–80
    after C-sections, 62, 185
    asthma and, 140
    blood sugar and, 118
    in breast milk, 200
    in complex carbohydrates, 109, 111
    as food for beneficial bacteria, 38–39
    food groups containing, ranking of, 78–79
    in infant formulas, 79–80, 211–212
    insoluble fibre, 78
    iron absorption and, 130
    microbiome and, 34–35, 77–83
    risk of atopic disease and, 235–238
    soluble fibre, 78
    in supplements, 219–220
fish, 94–99
    farmed fish, 148
    high-DHA fish, 98–99
    pollution of, 96–98
    wild vs. farmed, 96–97
fish oil. *See also* omega-3 fatty acids

DHA and, 95
from fish consumption, 94–99
risk of atopic disease and, 235–238
in supplements, 142–144, 219
Fleming, Alexander, 148
Florey, Howard, 149
folate (vitamin B9), 122–126
    food sources of, 126
    MTFHR mutation, 123–126
    neural tube development and, 123–124
folic acid, 124–125, 219
food additives, 85, 117
food allergies
    allergic rhinitis and, 23–24
    biggest effect on risk for, 233–243
    C-sections and, 183
    development of, 24–27
    fish oil and, 95, 142
    gestational diabetes and, 113, 127
    most common, 24
    prebiotic fibre and, 183
    probiotics and, 139–140
    treatment of, 139–140
foods. *See also* Mediterranean diet; organic and eco-products, benefits for babies
    choices, risk of atopic disease and, 238–239
    choline, sources of, 135–136
    "Clean Fifteen," 157
    cost of, 155–159
    DHA, sources for, 143
    "Dirty Dozen," 156–157
    eating the rainbow, 118
    from farmers' markets and independent farmers, 157
    as folate sources, 126
    foodborne pathogens, 48
    grow your own, 158
    healthy choices in, 220
    iodine, sources of, 133–134
    iron, sources of, 130–131
    junk foods, 107–108
    pesticides and, 151–155
    solid foods for babies, 34, 213–216
    sweet treats, 118–119
    vitamin E, sources of, 137
    for weaning, 214–216
    zinc, sources of, 132
formaldehyde, 165–167, 171, 173
formula-feeding

N

natural cleaning products, cosmetics and baby care products, 161–178. *See also* cleaning products; cosmetics
neural tubes, 122–123
New York State Department of Health, 164
non-heme iron, 130–131
nutrition. *See also* foods
    fats, good and bad, 85–105. *See also* fats and fatty acids
    feeding good bacteria, 77–83. *See also* bacteria; good bacteria
    health and, 2–4
    nutrients commonly deficient during pregnancy, 229–231
    risk of atopic disease and, 235–238
    sugar as cause of obesity and chronic disease, 107–120. *See also* sugar
    supplements, pregnancy and, 121–144. *See also* supplements
nuts
    ALA in, 94, 139
    allergies to, 24
    health benefits, 78, 80, 86–88, 90, 220
    introducing into babies' diets, 214–215
    vitamin E in, 137
    zinc in, 132

O

observational studies, 9–11
oestrogens, 212–213
olive oil, 80, 87–89, 118, 120, 137, 172, 220
Olkin, Ingram, 151
omega-3 fatty acids
    ALA, 94
    DHA, 94–96
    EPA, 94
    organic foods and, 150–151, 158
    pollution and, 96–99
    PUFAs, 91–96
    in supplements, 142–144
omega-6 fatty acids, 86–87, 90–96
organic and eco-products, benefits for babies, 147–159. *See also* cleaning products
    animal farming, antibiotics in, 147–149
    baby care products, 166–168, 176–178
    infant formulas, 213
    organic food, cost of, 155–159

organic food, is it healthier?, 149–155
overweight, 89, 112–113
oxytocin, 37, 203

P

palmitic acid, 103–104
palm oil, 99, 103–104
parabens, 162–163, 165–167, 171, 173
passive immunity, 199
peanut allergies, 139
penicillin, 148–149
perfumes. *See* essential oils; fragrances, artificial
personal care products, 165–166, 172–173
pesticides, 151–154, 219, 234–235
phthalates, 162, 165
pistachios, 90
pituitary glands, 183–184
plastics, BPA in, 43–44
pneumonia, 68
pollution
    indoor air pollution, 161–163
    seafood and, 96–99
polyunsaturated fats (PUFA), 86–87, 91–96
postpartum depression, 144
preeclampsia, 113, 127, 141
pregnancy. *See also* birth choices
    choline intake, 135
    cleaning products choice during, 162
    DHA, 98–99, 143
    essential oils during, 175
    fish oil and, 142–143
    folate supplements, 122–123
    hygiene hypothesis and, 48
    iodine intake, 133
    iron intake, 129
    mother's diet, effect on foetus of, 119–120
    mother's immune system during, 27
    nausea during, 133
    pesticides, effect on foetus, 151–152
    trans fats consumption, 105
    vitamin E intake, 137
    zinc intake, 131–132
Prevotella, 34
probiotics
    antibiotics and, 66, 69–74
    brain, effects on, 38
    BV, treatment of, 57–58

ABOUT THE AUTHORS

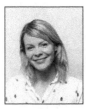 **MICHELLE HENNING** is a graduate of the Irish Institute of Nutrition & Health. Her articles have been featured in *WIRED Magazine*, *Pathways to Family Wellness*, *BabyCenter*, and many other outlets.

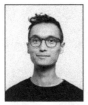 **DR. VICTOR HENNING** is an award-winning scientist, Fellow of the Royal Society of Arts, and founder of Mendeley, a leading scientific collaboration platform. He has published in peer-reviewed scientific journals and has been featured in the *New York Times* and *The Guardian*.

Michelle and Victor are lifelong allergy sufferers. They wanted their baby to grow up healthy, so they investigated the medical literature on how to prevent chronic illness. In this book, they share their research with other parents.

CPSIA information can be obtained
at www.ICGtesting.com
Printed in the USA
LVHW011158151220
674215LV00006B/441

9 781544 507798